LECTURE NOTES ON ENDOCRINOLOGY

Lecture Notes on
ENDOCRINOLOGY

RONALD F. FLETCHER
PhD, MD, FRCP

Consultant Physician
Dudley Road Hospital, Birmingham

Senior Clinical Lecturer
University of Birmingham

THIRD EDITION

BLACKWELL SCIENTIFIC PUBLICATIONS
OXFORD LONDON EDINBURGH
BOSTON MELBOURNE

In Memory of J R Squire

First published 1967
Second edition 1978
Reprinted 1979
Third edition 1982

Printed and
bound by
Billings Book Plan
Worcester

DISTRIBUTORS

USA
  Blackwell Mosby Book Distributors
  11830 Westline Industrial Drive
  St Louis, Missouri 63141

Canada
  Blackwell Mosby Book Distributors
  120 Melford Drive, Scarborough
  Ontario, M1B 2X4

Australia
  Blackwell Scientific Book Distributors
  214 Berkeley Street, Carlton
  Victoria 3053

British Library
Cataloguing in Publication Data

Fletcher, Ronald F.
  Lecture notes on endocrinology.—
    3rd ed.
  1. Endocrine glands—Diseases
  I. Title
  616.4   RC648

  ISBN 0-632-00842-3

Contents

Preface

This book is a guide to clinical endocrinology for medical students. The material presented covers the understanding, diagnosis and management of all the endocrine disorders likely to be met in everyday practice and consequently also much of what is required in the subject for diplomas in medicine and surgery.

For compactness, each gland is dealt with in turn and the emphasis is on the practical aspects. Most space is devoted to common disorders although others are mentioned and defined. Less attention is given to matters which are of little practical significance at present, despite their theoretical interest. Terminology is as simple as possible and eponyms, unless essential, are shown only as alternatives. For brevity the historical, embryological and comparative aspects of endocrinology have largely been omitted. Similarly, it has often been necessary to include only the conventional or most plausible doctrines without discussing the alternatives.

Methods of biochemical analysis and their clinical deployment are evolving quickly and local practice varies. Consequently, detailed instructions are not given but general indications and approximate reference ranges are included for the commoner tests. In practice, it is necessary to find out what assays are available, the recommended protocols and their interpretation, from the laboratories with which one is dealing.

In recommendations about treatment, well established preparations are preferred and the many commercial alternatives are not discussed. The suggestions for further reading at the end of each chapter consist mainly of recent books or reviews rather than publications of original research.

In the preparation of the earlier text I was helped by many colleagues but particularly Professor R. Hoffenberg. For this edition it is a pleasure to acknowledge the benefits of discussion with many colleagues but particularly the comments of Dr David Anderson. The errors and omissions are my own.

RONALD F. FLETCHER

Chapter 1
Introduction

ROLE OF ENDOCRINE SYSTEM

The role of the endocrine system is to act with the nervous system as the means whereby the function of the organism is controlled. The endocrine system has three distinguishing features. Firstly, its speed of response which is relatively slow, being in minutes to days in comparison with the fast responses of the nervous system. Secondly, its information is conveyed via hormones which are liberated into tissue fluids or the circulation. Thirdly, it is largely self-regulating. There are probably a number of links between the two nervous and endocrine systems but the hypothalamic/pituitary connection is of outstanding importance.

INTERNAL CONTROL

The ways in which the endocrine system is controlled are gradually being revealed. Three separate arrangements can be made out but as they are interrelated the overall organisation is highly complex.

1

Cyclical variations

There are many rhythmic variations in the endocrine system, mediated via the anterior pituitary. The monthly menstrual cycle is perhaps the most obvious and depends on interactions between the glands involved. Controlled more directly by the brain are the circadian rhythms which modulate the release of the anterior pituitary hormones during each twenty four hour period. The underlying neuronal activity is inherent but is continuously retimed by the alternation of light and dark and the associated periods of consciousness and sleep. This rhythm will adjust to a modification of the cycle, or a complete reversal as in shift work, but the adjustment takes several days. The main trends of variation in the plasma level of the anterior pituitary hormones under the influence of this circadian rhythm are shown in Fig. 1.1.

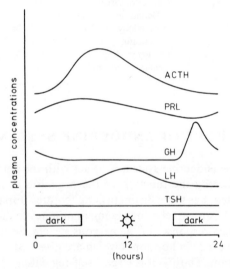

Fig. 1.1. Circadian rhythms of the plasma levels of some anterior pituitary hormones. The curves are smoothed and idealised. The scales are arbitrary and unrelated.

Response to environment

The release of cortisol and catecholamines in response to physical or emotional stress is well recognised but there are many other changes which may be important, for example after surgery. The intake of food releases gut hormones and insulin.

'Feed-back'

The self-regulation of the endocrine system is achieved by a number of 'feed-back' arrangements, many of considerable complexity. Both negative and positive feed-back are involved. Fig. 1.2 shows the essential features. The sensitivities and responses of the receptor apparatus at various parts of the loop are such that the system tends towards an equilibrium but in many instances the equilibrium point varies with circumstances. Most of the known feed-back loops involve the anterior pituitary and its target glands but the same considerations apply, for example, to the parathyroid glands, plasma calcium and bone.

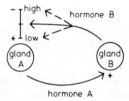

Fig. 1.2. A typical 'feed-back' loop. Gland 'A' liberates hormone 'A' which stimulates (+) gland 'B'. This releases hormone 'B' which modulates the liberation of hormone 'A'. The responsiveness of the receptor at gland 'A' can be moved up or down. The purpose of this arrangement is to control the plasma level of hormone 'B'.

Examples of these control arrangements will be found in many aspects of endocrine physiology and disease. Also, use is made of them frequently in endocrine investigation and treatment.

HORMONE RELEASE

Many hormones from the pituitary and other glands are released in sudden pulses at intervals of minutes or hours. As many hormones have a fast turnover in the circulation this means that their plasma levels may rise and fall rapidly over a few minutes which no doubt contributes to the difficulty of interpreting isolated measurements.

CIRCULATING HORMONES

The steroid and thyroid hormones are carried in the plasma largely bound to protein. Many proteins including albumin are involved but in particular there are several specific carrier globulins which have high affinities for their hormones. It is presumably the free hormone fraction which is in equilibrium with the cell hormone receptors and therefore biologically active. Total plasma concentrations may depend more on the concentrations or affinities of the carrier proteins than on anything else and may therefore give a misleading impression about tissue effects. Peptide hormones may be present in combinations of various molecular sizes and fragments of the larger polypeptides may be present also.

HORMONE ACTION

For the peptide hormones there are specific receptors on cell membranes, e.g. for hormones from the anterior pituitary, posterior pituitary and parathyroid. The activation of receptor sites by the arrival of these hormones releases (or suppresses) adenyl cyclase and the cyclic adenosine monophosphate (cAMP) produced then moves to other parts of the cell to activate protein kinases. The resulting reactions lead to the appropriate hormone effect. As the cAMP is the 'second messenger' mediating the action of many hormones it must be directed to its proper destination in the cell according to the nature of the stimulus, perhaps by passage along cellular structures related to specific receptors.

Steroid hormones pass through cell membranes and are bound to specific cytoplasmic receptors. The resulting complexes are translocated to the nucleus where they cause the transcription of specific messenger RNA's. These then move back into the cytoplasm where protein synthesis takes place.

Thyroid hormones enter cells and apparently have a fast action by activation of mitochondrial energy metabolism and a slow action on protein synthesis perhaps via nuclear receptors. The mode of action of insulin is not well understood but it reacts with surface receptors as well as entering cells.

HORMONE METABOLISM

In general, very little of any hormone which is synthesised exerts an action on the tissues and even the little that does is not necessarily destroyed in the process of doing so. Nearly all the mass of a hormone is degraded by systems quite independent of its site of action and the metabolic pathways vary with the individual hormones.

ENDOCRINE DISEASE

Definition

Many features of endocrine disorders result from an excess or a deficiency of a chemical which is present in normal health. The concentrations of hormones vary considerably in normal people so there can never be an exact dividing line between normal and abnormal endocrine function. Biochemical analysis in an individual can be related only to a reference range for a population and this restricts the value of tests in the borderline case. Fortunately, time will resolve the problems and without harm to the patient. Accurate diagnosis is particularly important because in most instances once treatment is started retesting is difficult or impossible. Unless treatment is urgent some confirmatory tests should be done even in obvious disease.

Aetiology

There is increasing evidence of genetic predisposition to endocrine disorders, particularly diabetes and thyroid disease, but the environmental triggers, if any, are uncertain. Atrophy of endocrine glands is relatively common and often autoimmune processes are involved but the primary fault is unknown. Similarly, gland-stimulating antibodies are important in Graves' disease but their initiation is obscure. Sometimes glands produce hormones in abnormal proportions. Disease may arise from a resistance to hormone action.

Endocrine glands form tumours readily but fortunately most of them are benign. The tumours may be non-functioning but many of them retain the capacity to synthesise the hormone(s) of the parent gland or cell type. However, the neoplastic tissue loses most or all of the normal feed-back modulation systems so that excess hormone secretion tends to occur.

CONCLUSION

Although it forms a coherent subject and it is easy to learn about it as such, endocrinology is linked with general medicine and gynaecology and should not be considered in isolation. Many endocrine diseases are eminently treatable so it is well worth while to be on the lookout for them.

FURTHER READING

VERHOEVEN G.F.M. & WILSON J.D. (1979). The syndromes of primary hormone resistance. *Metabolism,* **28,** 253.

WEITZMAN E.D. (1976). Circadian rhythms and episodic hormone secretion in man. *Annual Review of Medicine,* **27,** 225.

GENERAL REFERENCES

There are a number of books which can be consulted usefully on many endocrine topics. To avoid listing them at the end of every chapter, they are grouped here.

CLINICS IN ENDOCRINOLOGY AND METABOLISM (1973 et seq.). W.B. Saunders, London.

DEGROOT L.J. *et al* (1979). *Endocrinology (3 volumes)* Grune & Stratton, New York.

HALL R. *et al* (1980). *Fundamentals of Clinical Endocrinology.* (3rd Edition) Pitman, London.

MONTGOMERY D.A.D. & WELBOURN R.B. (1975). *Medical and Surgical Endocrinology,* Edward Arnold, London.

PINCHERA A. *et al* (Eds) (1980). *Autoimmune Aspects of Endocrine Disorders.* Academic Press, London.

WILLIAMS R.H. (Ed) (1980). *Textbook of Endocrinology (6th Edition).* W. B. Saunders, London.

Chapter 2
Pancreas and Carbohydrate

PANCREAS

The adult pancreas weighs between 50 and 70 g and lies behind the peritoneum with its head in the curve of the duodenum and its tail near the hilum of the spleen. Most of the pancreas is concerned with its exocrine function, the production of pancreatic secretion for intestinal digestion. The endocrine portion is only 1–2% of the gland by weight and consists of about 2 million *Islets of Langerhans*. These are highly vascularised areas ranging in size from a few cells to nodules 300 μm across.

In the islets three main cell types have been identified so far:

Cell type	Proportion of Islet %	Hormone produced
B	80	Insulin
A	15	Glucagon
D	?	Somatostatin

The Islet has a complex internal organisation of unknown purpose. The outer layers of cells contain glucagon, with a few cells containing

7

Chapter 2

somatostatin; the core of the islet consists of insulin containing cells (Fig. 2.1).

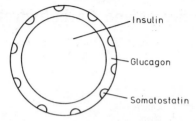

FIG. 2.1. The distribution of some of the hormone secreting cells of the Islet of Langerhans implying a complex internal organisation.

INSULIN

The B cells synthesise a single chain polypeptide called pro-insulin (Fig. 2.2). This molecule is cleaved to yield insulin, and 'C' peptide; all three

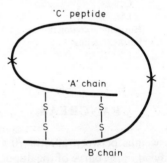

FIG. 2.2. The molecule of pro-insulin. Cleavage occurs at the positions indicated by the two crosses to release insulin (A and B chain with two disulphide bridges) and 'C'-peptide.

substances are released into the circulation. Insulin contains an 'A' peptide chain of 21 amino acids and a 'B' chain of 30 amino acids joined by two di-sulphide bridges. The beef and pork insulins used in treatment differ from human insulin in respect of three and one amino acids respectively. This makes them immunologically distinct, but has little effect on their potency in man.

Release

The rate of synthesis and release of insulin is determined largely by the level of blood glucose, a rise in glucose causing a rise in insulin. Many other factors can cause insulin release including amino acids, some lipids, vagal stimulation and glucagon. Probably of more physiological importance is the effect of glucose absorption from the intestine which produces a greater insulin release than would be expected from the rise in blood glucose alone (Fig. 2.3). This effect is thought to be mediated by gut hormones.

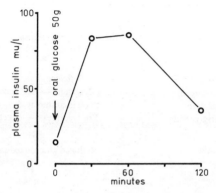

FIG. 2.3. A normal response of plasma insulin to oral glucose.

Insulin in plasma

The concentration of insulin in normal plasma varies over the wide range of 10 to 50 mu/l depending on the state of absorption. Such low concentrations can be measured routinely only by immunoassay but the insulin activity in the plasma as measured by bioassay does not necessarily equate with the immunoreactive insulin.

Metabolism

Insulin is removed rapidly from the plasma with a half-life of about four minutes. It is disposed of by degradation in many tissues, particularly the liver and kidney.

Insulin action

The most important tissues on which insulin has a direct action are the liver, muscle (including heart) and adipose tissue. Nearly all tissues are affected in some way but in many the effects are secondary. In many tissues there are specific receptors for insulin on the cell membranes but it seems that insulin may also penetrate the cell. The major action of insulin is to permit the penetration of glucose and other closely similar sugars into cells but some of the actions are additional to and independent of glucose penetration (Table 2.1). Insulin has no effect on the intestinal or renal handling of glucose.

TABLE 2.1. Effects of Insulin

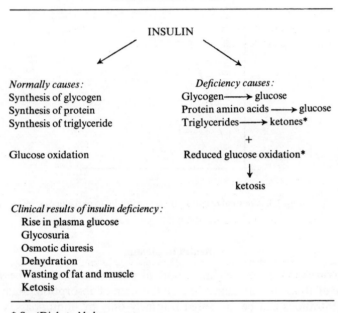

INSULIN

Normally causes:
Synthesis of glycogen
Synthesis of protein
Synthesis of triglyceride

Glucose oxidation

Deficiency causes:
Glycogen⟶glucose
Protein amino acids ⟶ glucose
Triglycerides⟶ketones*
+
Reduced glucose oxidation*
↓
ketosis

Clinical results of insulin deficiency:
Rise in plasma glucose
Glycosuria
Osmotic diuresis
Dehydration
Wasting of fat and muscle
Ketosis

* See 'Diabetes' below

GLUCAGON

This is a single chain polypeptide of known structure containing 29 amino acids; it can be measured by immunoassay. Glucagon stimulates the secretion of insulin but paradoxically its major metabolic effect is to raise plasma glucose by stimulating glycogenolysis in the liver. Many other effects have been demonstrated but the role of glucagon in human physiology and pathology remains uncertain. It seems that the presence of glucagon is not essential for the genesis of diabetes mellitus.

CARBOHYDRATE METABOLISM

In the average British diet about 45% of the calories are derived from carbohydrate and most adults take between 100 and 300 g per day. The carbohydrate is mostly starch, sucrose, cane and beet sugar and lactose (milk) but these are digested in the small intestinal lumen and mucosa so that only monosaccharides are absorbed, the ratios being approximately glucose 80%, fructose 15% and galactose 5%. The fructose and galactose are extracted by the liver, even in the absence of insulin, and enter the glucose and glycogen metabolic pathways. In clinical practice only glucose is significant; it has not been possible to use other sugars in the management of diabetes.

In the normal person, after food the plasma glucose is controlled by insulin release and subsequent disposal of glucose into tissues. During prolonged starvation the plasma glucose is always maintained. At first, this is done by glycogenolysis in the liver and muscles but this store is soon exhausted and then glucose has to be synthesised from amino acids as it cannot be made from fatty acids.

Many factors, including hormones, alter carbohydrate metabolism in complex ways. An excess of glucocorticoid and growth hormone tends to diminish carbohydrate tolerance perhaps by interference with the action of insulin. Glucocorticoid deficiency increases insulin action. Glucagon and adrenaline tend to raise plasma glucose by promoting glycogenolysis.

KETONE METABOLISM

The oxidation of fatty acids leads to the production of acetyl CoA. Normally, this:

1. Joins with oxaloacetate and enters the Krebs cycle to release energy.
2. Condenses to form acetoacetyl CoA and thus ketone bodies.

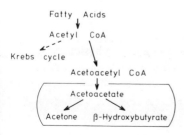

FIG. 2.4. Ketone production in diabetes. Insulin lack accelerates fatty acid oxidation but restricts the disposal of acetyl CoA through the Krebs cycle. The ketones are bracketed.

In diabetes when carbohydrate utilisation is defective there is an increased oxidation of fatty acid and at the same time a deficient supply of oxaloacetate so that the excess acetyl CoA is deflected into the production of ketones (Fig. 2.4). Ketone bodies can be oxidised in muscle but when production is high the disposal system is overloaded and ketones accumulate. Starvation alone will increase ketone production sufficiently to produce positive urine tests.

HYPOGLYCAEMIA

This may occur in many circumstances but except with insulin treatment plasma levels low enough to cause symptoms (i.e. below about 2.5 mmol/l)* are uncommon. Nearly all hypoglycaemic states are intermittent and depend on the pattern of food intake, the lowest levels occurring two hours or more after the last meal. The symptoms are a mixture of direct effects of glucose lack on the brain ('neuroglucopenia') and the results of adrenaline release. The former tend to produce irritability, agitation, confusion and sleepiness while the latter are characterised by nervousness, weakness, palpitations, hunger, fear and sweating. However, the pattern of symptoms is very variable and may depend on the speed of fall of the plasma glucose as well as age and chronicity. There may well be considerable difficulty in diagnosis.

Causes

A full list of known causes of hypoglycaemia is large; the commoner types are:

> Primary pancreatic
> Toxic
> Reactive
> Hepatic
> Endocrine
> Childhood forms

Primary pancreatic
This is due to insulin secreting tissue escaping from physiological control. Usually there is an insulinoma which is a small, benign adenoma of islet tissue but which may rarely be multiple ('microadenomatosis') or malignant.

* 45 mg/100 ml

The diagnosis may be difficult because the symptoms are variable. The patients are usually young adults or middle aged; about half have episodes of unconsciousness or fits and may be thought to be epileptic. Other presentations may include episodes of confusion, weakness, sweating, amnesia and various psychiatric syndromes. Intermittent or focal neurological abnormalities may be present. A tendency for the episodes to occur some hours after food is a useful clue and the patient may have noticed that food helps the symptoms.

Management at first is by regular meals and glucose supplements as necessary. Definitive treatment is by excision but pre-operative localisation of the tumour is difficult. Otherwise, the drug diazoxide or the more toxic streptozotocin may be helpful.

Toxic
The commonest cause is relative overdosage of injected insulin due to changing needs, error or malice (see Chapter 4). Long acting sulphonylureas and also alcohol (by inhibiting gluconeogenesis) may be causes.

Reactive
In some persons the insulin response to food is delayed and exaggerated leading to hypoglycaemia a few hours after a meal. Emotional or prediabetic individuals are particularly liable to this condition. The symptoms are usually mild. A similar syndrome may occur after partial gastrectomy.

Hepatic
Any type of liver disease may be associated with hypoglycaemia but there is no correlation between the relative severity of the two conditions and the cause of the relationship is uncertain.

Endocrine
Hypopituitarism and hypoadrenalism may be associated with hypoglycaemia.

Childhood
Hypoglycaemia in children may arise from causes which do not occur in adults. In 'neonatal hypoglycaemia' the normal fall in plasma glucose at that time is unduly prolonged, for no apparent reason. Infants born to diabetic mothers may have some degree of islet overactivity with low plasma glucose for several days. Hypoglycaemia of childhood may have no detectable cause but a similar condition is produced by leucine sensitivity, galactosaemia and glycogen storage disease.

Rare causes of hypoglycaemia include the release of substances with 'insulin-like-activity' from malignant tumours (see Chapter 13).

Diagnosis

In adults, it is desirable to establish the diagnosis by Whipple's triad of: symptoms induced by fasting, simultaneous demonstration of hypo-glycaemia (i.e. plasma glucose less than 2.5 mmol/l) and the relief of symptoms by glucose. The diagnosis of insulinoma can be established by inducing these features after fasting, if necessary for as long as 72 h. The demonstration of an inappropriately high plasma insulin com-pared with the plasma glucose at that time is further strong evidence for an insulin secreting tumour.

Many other tests have been described (e.g. using the administration of tolbutamide, glucagon, leucine or fish insulin) but some of them are potentially dangerous and they add little to what can be learnt from observations following a glucose load or during fasting. In children, complex tests may be necessary.

HORMONE SECRETING TUMOURS OF THE PANCREAS

These are of two main types. Carcinomas of the pancreas, arising presumably from duct epithelium, are common but mostly do not seem to secrete hormones. Sometimes, such tumours are the site of 'ectopic hormone production' (see Chapter 13). The well known association between peripheral venous thrombosis and early carcinoma of the pan-creas does raise the possibility of a humoral relationship but no more is known. Pancreatic tumours arising from endocrine tissue usually are benign but have the capacity to secrete the appropriate hormone out-side physiological control; malignant change may occur. Three specific tumours are recognised:

Insulinoma
This is described above.

Gastrinoma
These tumours, which may be single or multiple, cause the Zollinger–Ellison syndrome. The persistent secretion of large amounts of gastrin causes excessive production of gastric acid leading to severe recurrent ulceration of the upper gastrointestinal tract. Diarrhoea is common

and malabsorption may occur. The diagnosis is suggested by the finding of a high and continuous secretion of gastric juice and acid, and is confirmed by raised levels of plasma gastrin. Treatment is by resection of the secreting tumour.

Glucagonoma

This rare tumour causes a bizarre syndrome comprising mild diabetes, weight loss, glossitis, stomatitis and necrotising cutaneous erythema. Diagnosis is by finding a raised level of plasma glucagon and treatment is by excision.

FURTHER READING

CORNBLATH, M. & SCHWARTZ, R. (1976). *Disorders of Carbohydrate Metabolism in Infancy*, (2nd Edition), W.B. Saunders, London.

FAJANS, S.S. & FLOYD, J.C. (1976). Fasting hypoglycemia in adults. *New England Journal of Medicine*, **294**, 766.

FELIG, P., *et al* (1979). Hormonal interactions in the regulation of blood glucose. *Recent Progress in Hormone Research*, **35**, 501.

GRIMELIUS, L. & WILANDER, E. (1980). Silver Stains in the study of endocrine cells of the gut and pancreas. *Investigative and Cell Pathology*, **3**, 3.

MODLIN, I.M. (1979). Endocrine tumors of the pancreas. *Surgery, Gynecology and Obstetrics*, **149**, 751.

Chapter 3
Diabetes Mellitus—Clinical

DEFINITION

There is no agreed exact definition of diabetes. One approach is to consider only the blood glucose levels after a standard glucose load and use the upper limits of normality as laid down by the British Diabetic Association (see below). This is simple but will diagnose as diabetic a number of persons, particularly amongst the elderly, who have no symptoms at the time and who will never develop symptoms or complications of diabetes. There is disagreement also as to whether an increased level under a glucose load only will suffice. In practice, most patients are plainly diabetic with symptoms and/or complications and there is no problem in diagnosis but the counselling and management of the patient with borderline changes may be difficult.

PRESENTATION

The clinical picture of primary diabetes mellitus is very variable, ranging from years of trivial glycosuria to death from ketoacidosis in a few

16

weeks. The illness has two main forms, namely *Early-onset* (juvenile onset or type I) and *Late-onset* (adult or maturity onset, or type II). (Table 3.1). This classification is a general guide only and exceptions occur. An alternative classification is '*Insulin Dependent Diabetes*' (IDD) and '*Non-insulin Dependent Diabetes*' (NIDD). Diabetes may be latent in that carbohydrate tolerance is lost only under stress (see below).

Sometimes the patients presenting symptoms such as abdominal pain, weakness, loss of weight, cramp or breathlessness do not immediately suggest diabetes. Thirst and polyuria may be regarded by the patient as being of no significance and admitted to only in response to a direct question. In late-onset diabetes delay in diagnosis is unfortunate but in early-onset diabetes it can be disastrous. Routine urine testing is essential in clinical practice.

Other uncommon forms of primary diabetes occur. There is a Maturity Onset Diabetes of the Young (MODY) and also the combination of Diabetes Insipidus, Diabetes Mellitus, Optic Atrophy and Deafness (DIDMOAD). There is an association between diabetes and thyroid disease, Addison's disease, pernicious anaemia and some uncommon hereditary syndromes.

Rarely, secondary diabetes may follow pancreatic damage from inflammation, haemochromatosis, tumour or surgery.

TABLE 3.1. Features of types of diabetes.

Early-onset (type I) (i.e. juvenile, under 30 years of age)	Late-onset (type II) (i.e. 'maturity' or adult i.e. over 30 years of age)
Thin	Usually obese
Weight loss marked	Weight loss slight
Pruritus unusual	Pruritus common
Ill: nausea, vomiting	Mild illness only
Ketosis usually present	Ketosis absent
Usually insulin dependent	Usually non-insulin dependent
Thirst and polyuria	Thirst and polyuria

SYMPTOMS AND SIGNS

Apart from changes in vision (see below) *hyperglycaemia* in itself produces no definite symptoms and therefore cannot be detected by the individual. The leakage of glucose into the urine when the plasma level exceeds about 10 mmol/l causes an osmotic diuresis. This polyuria leads to dehydration perceived as thirst which the patient relieves by drinking extra fluid i.e. *polydipsia*. Polyuria and polydipsia are the cardinal symptoms of diabetes.

In *early-onset* diabetes the history is usually of a few weeks duration only. The thirst and polyuria are soon joined by more severe symptoms of increasing tiredness, anorexia and weight loss. Later there may be cramps, apparent breathlessness, nausea, vomiting and abdominal pain, the latter particularly in children. Sometimes, if untreated, the patient may become drowsy or even comatose from ketoacidosis. On examination the patient is likely to be thin and may be dehydrated. Features of ketoacidosis (see below) may be present. Diabetic complications are unlikely to be found but there may be a precipitating cause such as an infection.

In *late-onset* diabetes the history is likely to be of several months duration. There may be some degree of general debility and a varying degree of weight loss. Pruritus vulvae or balanitis is common. On examination, the majority of patients will be obese but some are not. Apart from inflammation of the vulva or foreskin from secondary infection, specific signs are likely to be absent except for absent ankle reflexes. Occasionally, diabetic complications are observed on presentation implying a longstanding but unrecognised diabetic state.

COMPLICATIONS

In many respects the complications of diabetes are the most important aspect of the disease as they are the major source of discomfort and hazard to the patients; many are resistant to treatment.

The complications may be grouped as:

Biochemical
Microvascular
Macrovascular
Neurological
Miscellaneous

The biochemical complications may arise at any time in the course of diabetes and may indeed be part of the presentation. They are less common in the adult-onset form. The other complications occur in relation to the duration of the diabetes with wide individual differences. The time scale is 10 to 50 years so that newly diagnosed early-onset diabetics are unlikely to have vascular complications whereas those who have been on insulin for forty years will probably have vascular changes. In late-onset non-insulin dependent diabetes vascular complications occur also, but because of the late age of onset many patients do not have a remaining life span long enough for complications to develop. It is possible that there are mild variants of diabetes which do not carry the risk of complications but this is unproven.

Biochemical

If diabetes escapes from control with a high and rising plasma glucose two patterns of biochemical disorder may occur.

Ketoacidosis (diabetic coma and precoma)

This may be a presenting feature of insulin-dependent diabetes but is seen more commonly as an incident during treatment. There may be a precipitating factor such as stress from an infection but just as often no cause can be found. In the early stages there is usually nausea and anorexia. Sometimes insulin doses are reduced or omitted under the erroneous impression that this is appropriate when food cannot be taken. Over a few days or even less there is increasing thirst and polyuria; malaise, anorexia, vomiting and often abdominal pain. The patient becomes drowsy or even unconscious.

On examination there is dehydration with a hot dry skin and dry tongue. The eyes are sunken and the pulse is fast with a low blood pressure. The respiration is increased in amplitude and rate (Kussmaul 'air hunger') and the sweet smell of acetone can be detected on the patient's breath by those with sensitive noses. Biochemical tests confirm the diagnosis. The urine will contain at least 2% glucose and heavy ketonuria will be present. In the plasma the expected findings would be:

Glucose > 20 mmol/l (> 360 mg/100 ml)
Bicarbonate < 10 mmol/l
P_{CO_2} < 4 KPa (< 30 mmHg)
pH < 7.2

The blood urea is likely to be raised; plasma potassium may be normal or raised.

Hyperosmolar non-ketotic coma and precoma

This is less common than ketoacidosis but not rare. It arises usually in obese late-onset diabetics whose disease has been mild or undiagnosed. The clinical features are similar to those described above in so far as dehydration and drowsiness are concerned but acidosis is absent and therefore respiration is normal. In the urine, ketones are absent or present only in small amounts. The plasma glucose is very high (hence the hyperosmolar state) and the plasma sodium may be raised also.

(Lactic acidosis may occur in diabetics but is much less common now phenformin is not used; see under treatment, below).

Microvascular

The microvascular changes are specific to diabetes. Probably many organs are affected but symptoms or signs arise from the retinae, glomerulae, myocardium and perhaps some nerves.

Retinopathy

Is a common condition and is likely to be present in the majority of patients who have been diabetic for more than 15 years. The retinopathy is usually slight and symptomless and may progress only slowly but this is not always the case and the more extensive forms endanger sight. Diabetic retinopathy is now the commonest single cause of blindness in the UK in persons under 65 years of age.

Features of diabetic retinopathy

Five components can be distinguished. They may occur independently but more commonly increase together. The extent of the lesions varies widely from a few dots and exudates (background retinopathy) to extensive destruction.

a) Haemorrhages. These may be tiny red 'dots' indistinguishable from microaneurysms (see below) or larger 'blot' haemorrhages.

b) New vessel formation. This occurs at first as a few new capillaries going on to extensive patches of new vessels.

c) Vascular involvement. The arteries and arterioles show irregularity or occlusion of the lumen while the veins show dilatation and beading. The arterioles develop saccular microaneurysms which appear as small red dots.

d) Exudates. Deposits of lipid which are pale yellow with sharp lobulated outlines. They may form cuffs around blood vessels.

e) Proliferative retinopathy. In the more severe or later forms haemorrhage and new vessel formation begins to extend forward into the vitreous with the addition of fibrous tissue and sometimes retinal detachment.

Other features may be seen. Nearby lesions can cause macular oedema with reduction of visual acuity. Vascular occlusions lead to white patches with indistinct edges due to axonal degeneration but this appearance is not specific to diabetes and may be present in hypertension also.

Nephropathy
Vascular changes in the glomerular tufts in diabetics are common (see Pathology, below). The changes are symptomless in the early stages and are revealed only by a moderate proteinuria. Usually, this is all that happens and causes no trouble but in a proportion of patients there is progressive renal damage leading to uraemia. Oedema may occur but a true nephrotic syndrome is rare.

Macrovascular

The atheroma of large arteries and the common consequences of vascular occlusion (myocardial infarction, cerebral thrombosis and ischaemia of the legs) in diabetics is much the same as in non-diabetics. However, in diabetics the lesions tend to be extensive, affect smaller vessels as well and tend to occur at an earlier age. This latter feature accounts for much of the increased mortality in diabetics particularly from myocardial infarction. In addition, diabetics are liable to myocardial damage from microvascular disease.

Neurological

Peripheral nerves and the autonomic system may be affected but the central nervous system escapes.

Peripheral neuropathy
This is typically sensory and symmetrical. It is common but often asymptomatic, being revealed only by a loss of tendon reflexes and vibration sense. It is much more marked in the legs than in the arms. In more severe degree, numbness and paraesthesia in the feet may be troublesome and anaesthesia can be dangerous as unnoticed trauma may occur. Sometimes the condition causes severe pain. Rarely, there may be cranial nerve lesions and isolated peripheral nerve damage which may be sensory, motor or mixed. Charcot's joints and amyotrophy may occur.

Autonomic neuropathy
Autonomic neuropathy is common also but only on testing because it is less likely to cause symptoms. There may be pupillary abnormalities,

bladder disturbances, changes in sweating and loss of vasomotor reflexes. 'Diabetic diarrhoea', an unusual but troublesome complaint, is due probably to an autonomic neuropathy of the gut.

Miscellaneous

'Diabetic feet'
These present a special problem. Usually the primary lesions are ischaemic with gangrene of one or more toes due to occlusion of relatively small arteries in the feet. Sometimes the block is femoral with more extensive ischaemia or gangrene. Secondary infection may be troublesome. The role of neuropathy is less clear but blisters or ulcers may follow unnoticed trauma.

Infections
Diabetics are said to be unduly susceptible to infections but this is rarely a problem except in respect of the skin and urinary tract. A carbuncle is a classic but unusual mode of presentation; sepsis may unmask latent diabetes.

Cataracts
These are common in diabetics and occur at an earlier age than in non-diabetics. The usual appearances are of peripheral radial linear streaks or scattered dots.

Sexual function
Many middle-aged diabetic men complain of erectile impotence. It is proposed that the cause is autonomic neuropathy but this is unproven. Any equivalent loss of sexual function in women appears to be unrecorded but a failure of ability to reach orgasm would be expected. Fertility, in both sexes, and menstrual regularity is maintained.

Skin
The only skin lesion virtually specific to diabetes is *necrobiosis lipoidica diabeticorum*. It occurs most commonly in women of early middle age and is localised to the shins. There are papules going on to form pink and yellow plaques which may ulcerate but later heal. The histology is distinctive.

Plasma lipids
The level of the plasma cholesterol and triglycerides, particularly in the pre-β-lipoproteins, tends to rise in untreated diabetes. Rarely, uncon-

trolled diabetes is accompanied by milky plasma due to chylomicrons. Eruptive xanthomas may occur and the retinal vessels are pale (lipaemia retinalis).

AETIOLOGY

In primary diabetes there is no obvious cause but a number of factors have been implicated. There may be associated acromegaly or Cushing's syndrome.

Genetic

There is certainly some degree of hereditary disposition. In identical twins concordance for late-onset diabetes is almost complete but for early-onset diabetes the association is much weaker. Early-onset insulin dependent diabetes has a positive association with Histocompatability Leucocyte Antigen (HLA) loci DR3 and DR4. There is no HLA association with late-onset diabetes but despite this the condition is more strongly familial. The children of diabetics have an increased incidence of the disease; the exact risk is uncertain but is probably about three times that in other children. The sex ratio of diabetes tends to change with time—at present in the UK men and women are equally likely to be affected.

Infections

There are peaks of incidence of early-onset diabetes at ages 12 and 20 years and during the autumn and spring. Perhaps this is related to an increased incidence of certain virus infections causing an 'isletitis'.

Stress

Physical stress may induce a diabetic state. Any major physical trauma such as severe accident, burns, surgery or myocardial infarction impairs insulin release. Pregnancy (gestational diabetes) or the administration of corticosteroids can have a similar effect on the plasma glucose although the mediation may be different. In most patients carbohydrate tolerance is restored as and when the stress passes off but occasionally the diabetes persists. This may raise medico-legal problems after accidents.

Autoimmunity

Many recently diagnosed insulin-dependent diabetics have circulating islet tissue antibodies but they tend to disappear with time, perhaps as the islets are destroyed. Some other conditions related to auto-immunity, such as thyroid disease, pernicious anaemia and Addison's disease have an increased incidence in diabetes.

Diet

There is no established relationship between diet and the development of diabetes. It is unlikely to be relevant in the early-onset patient but in late-onset diabetes there is room for speculation. A high proportion of carbohydrate in the diet is in itself probably innocuous but refined sugar, particularly in the large amounts consumed in this country, might be harmful.

Obesity

Obese persons tend to have raised levels of plasma insulin and to be relatively insulin resistant. Why a few obese persons should then go on, perhaps after many years of obesity, to become diabetic is uncertain but there is no doubt that the majority of late-onset diabetics are overweight. In most such patients calorie restrictions will lower plasma glucose, even to normal.

Insulin production

The relationship between diabetes and insulin production is complex. In the early-onset ketotic diabetic there is undoubtedly a failure of insulin production and the plasma insulin is low or absent. In the obese late-onset non-ketotic diabetic the plasma insulin is normal or even raised and responds to a carbohydrate load. Presumably there is some factor which prevents its effective action and various theories have been proposed. However, exogenous insulin or increased insulin re-lease as a result of sulphonylurea treatment (see below) are effective and control the diabetic state.

Epidemiology

Despite the various factors discussed diabetes occurs in 1–2% of the population in many countries, cultures and historical periods.

PATHOLOGY

The pancreas in many insulin-dependent diabetics shows histological changes in the islets including reduction in mass, fibrosis, hyalinisation and lymphocytic infiltration, but the significance of these findings is uncertain. Microvascular complications are characterised particularly by a thickening of the basement membrane. It has been postulated that this is an underlying pathological fault which precedes a failure of carbohydrate tolerance but most present evidence indicates that the vascular changes are secondary to the diabetic condition. In the retina the most striking lesion is the microaneurysm. In the kidney the appearances in the glomerular tufts are described as nodular (Kimmelstiel-Wilson), diffuse or exudative, all tending to lead to glomerular hyalinisation. In diabetic neuropathy the peripheral nerves show segmental demyelination as well as cell loss in dorsal root ganglia and anterior horns. Axonal loss occurs also. Microvascular disease in relation to peripheral nerves may be important.

DIAGNOSIS

Certain tests and observations are crucial in diagnosis and treatment.

Glycosuria

Typical diabetic urine is copious because of the osmotic diuresis due to glucose, pale because the pigments are diluted in a large volume, and of high specific gravity because of the presence of glucose.

Glycosuria is best detected by a 'stick' test. Many are available either for glucose alone or in various combinations with other tests. The stick tests employ a specific glucose oxidase reaction so that false positives are rare. However, they are very sensitive and detect degrees of glycosuria which are insignificant so that they must be followed by other tests for diagnosis. Glycosuria can be quantitated with 'Diastix' (Ames Co.) which is now recommended in place of the older less convenient 'Clinitest'. *N.B.* Ketones interfere with the reaction so that false low readings may be obtained in ketoacidosis.

Ketonuria

Stick tests alone or in combination are satisfactory for screening and can give an approximate quantitation. These are sensitive and give positive reactions to the ketosis induced by starvation.

Plasma glucose

One of the specific glucose oxidase methods should be used for the biochemical estimation. If venous blood is taken, it must be mixed at once with a suitable inhibitor, such as fluoride, to prevent glycolysis. Levels quoted here are for capillary blood—those for venous blood are about 10% lower but this difference is not significant in practice. Usually whole blood is analysed but if serum or plasma is used the result is again slightly lower. There are 'stick' methods for use on blood; some may be used with reflectance meters to give a more accurate estimate. They are particularly useful in the ward or for home monitoring. The sticks deteriorate on exposure to air so careful storage is necessary and old ones should be discarded.

Glucose tolerance test (GTT)

This is a valuable test but not of good reproducibility even when carried out with the precautions described below. The patient should take normal exercise and an unrestricted diet for at least three days before the test. After a twelve hour overnight fast the patient sits quietly for half an hour. Smoking is forbidden. Specimens of blood and urine are collected and the patient drinks 250 ml of water, with a little flavouring if desired, containing 50 g of glucose. The usual practice in the USA is to give 100 g but this makes little difference to the interpretation of the test. For children, 1.75 g/kg body weight may be used. The patient then rests, without smoking or eating for two hours while blood and urine specimens are collected every 30 min.

Interpretation of results

The conventional upper limits of normal for a GTT are shown in Fig. 3.1. The significance of various findings are as follows:

1. Glycosuria with a GTT curve within normal limits:
   Renal glycosuria of no diabetic significance.
2. Ketonuria with normal blood glucose:
   Not diabetes—probably due to starvation.
3. High random blood glucose, e.g. more than 15 mmol/l* particularly if with ketonuria:
   Definite diabetes—a GTT is unnecessary.

* 270 mg/100 ml.

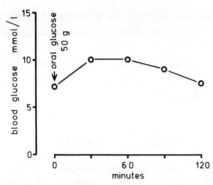

Fig. 3.1. The *upper* limit of normal during a standard oral glucose tolerance test. Capillary blood, true glucose method.

4. Interpretation of GTT.
   a) Blood glucose above normal throughout:
      Diabetes.
   b) Normal fasting level but blood glucose above normal during rest of test and at two hours:
      Probably diabetes (but some would disagree).
   c) Normal blood glucose fasting and after two hours, but raised levels between. This is called a 'lag storage curve' and may occur in various circumstances, e.g. after gastric surgery:
      Probably of no diabetic significance.
5. These criteria are reasonably reliable in patients under 60 years of age, however slight degrees of carbohydrate intolerance of doubtful significance become more common with advancing age. With borderline abnormalities retesting and further observation may be necessary.

NATURAL HISTORY OF DIABETES

For many patients the diagnosis is obvious and permanent but there are exceptions. Any stress may impede insulin release. In some individuals pregnancy and treatment with corticosteroids or diuretics may cause a transient diabetes. Even apparently established diabetes may be surprisingly phasic so that some patients have episodes of insulin dependence with later almost normal carbohydrate tolerance. The natural history of such patients is poorly understood.

The life expectancy in diabetes is somewhat reduced but is changing and difficult to summarize because it is related to the age at onset and to insulin dependence. The elderly non-insulin dependent diabetic can expect a life span little different from that of the non-diabetic, particularly if obesity is corrected, but the twenty year old male insulin taker, for example, has a life expectancy of 30–40 years compared with 50 years for the non-diabetic.

FURTHER READING

JEANRENAUD, B. (1979). Insulin and obesity. *Diabetologia*, **17**, 133.

KEEN, H. & JARRETT, J. (Eds.) (1975). *Complications of Diabetes*, Edward Arnold, London.

REPORT etc. (1976). Ten-year follow-up report on the Birmingham diabetes survey of 1961. *British Medical Journal*, **2**, 35.

(See also end of Chapter 4).

Chapter 4
Diabetes Mellitus—Treatment

INTRODUCTION

The control of diabetes is simple in theory but often difficult in practice. The obvious objective of normalizing the blood glucose is elusive, particularly in the insulin-dependent patient. There are two main problems in deciding on a suitable philosophy of treatment.

29

1. It is still not certain that complications can be prevented by good control. The patients know this so that the clinician's attitude and advice is weakened.

2. The care needed to achieve even reasonable control is beyond the determination or capabilities of many patients. Consequently, treatment is a series of compromises to retain the patient's co-operation, without which nothing can be achieved. The clinician has to devise a scheme of treatment which will give the best control possible in the circumstances. Particular emphasis is placed on the relief of diabetic symptoms, good control in the young patient (even if only to reduce the risk of ketoacidosis), and good control in the patient with advancing complications.

Management always involves several interrelated topics:

Diet
Oral hypoglycaemic drugs
Insulin
Education
Treatment of complications
Organisation of services

DIET

The treatment of diabetes always requires some change, but dietary habits are so ingrained that it may be difficult to achieve. Attention to certain details increases the chance of success:

1. Consider the patient's usual dietary habits, preferences, allergies and religious constraints, then recommend as few changes as are likely to be satisfactory.

2. Dietary advice must be appropriate to individual circumstances, e.g. not beyond the patient's finances and fitting in with his/her pattern of work and cooking facilities.

3. Try to explain the nature and purpose of the diet, and provide some written instructions for all except the simplest diet. Diet prescriptions should be treated like drug prescriptions with review and revision as appropriate.

The services of a qualified dietician are most valuable but often the doctor will have to manage without.

General principles of diabetic diet prescriptions
Opinions on diabetic diets are changing and recently the British Diabetic Association have set out new guidelines.

It is considered that overall calorie intake is more important than carbohydrate intake. Carbohydrate should provide 55% of total calories and should be taken in the form of foods such as bread, potatoes, cereals etc., as high in fibre as possible. Refined carbohydrates (e.g. sugar) should be used only in emergencies.

Fats should provide not more than 35% of total calories with a trend away from saturated fats (e.g. dairy products) towards polyunsaturated fats. It is doubtful whether cholestrol intake should be restricted but some recommend such a change. Although conclusive evidence is lacking, a reduction in salt intake is prudent. The diet should be adequate in proteins, vitamins and minerals.

Unless contraindicated medically, alcohol may be taken in moderate amounts provided allowance is made for the calories consumed. Special diabetic beers and processed goods are expensive and unnecessary. Saccharine may be used.

Specific diets

Diets for diabetics are of three main kinds.

Low calorie

Weight reduction by calorie restriction is the most important treatment for the obese late-onset diabetic. The principles are the same as for the non-diabetic obese person and are set out in Chapter 5.

Restricted calorie

The non-obese late-onset diabetic needs modest calorie restriction coupled with the elimination of refined sugar, along the lines of the general principles above.

Controlled carbohydrate

These diets are a necessary accompaniment of insulin therapy. The total carbohydrate intake is likely to be between 120 and 250 g/day depending on the patient's physique, work and need to gain or lose weight. A 10 g exchange system is used. In this, the patient is taught various 10 g rations of carbohydrate, e.g.

>Half a thick slice of bread
>One small boiled potato
>One medium apple
>Half a pint of beer, etc.

The diet prescription is set out for so many g of carbohydrate a day, distributed at different meals to take account of the patient's preferences and pattern of work. A typical prescription might be:

Breakfast	30 g
Mid morning	10 g
Lunch	50 g
Tea	30 g
Supper	50 g
Evening	10 g (Total 180 g)

The carbohydrate quantities at each meal are made up from the list of exchanges in any way the patient wishes and can be varied from day to day. Non-carbohydrate foods can be taken as necessary to make up a balanced and nutritious diet, and to adjust body weight. Variations in the total carbohydrate intake may be needed to meet special circumstances such as growth, pregnancy or change of job. As the insulin type and dose are usually the same each day it is important that the carbohydrate prescription is adhered to at each meal to avoid imbalance between carbohydrate and insulin. Changing insulin dose is no use unless the carbohydrate intake is regular. Some diabetics refuse to adhere to a diet, but this renders good diabetic control impossible.

ORAL HYPOGLYCAEMIC DRUGS

Sulphonylureas

This is the only group now in general use. They act by augmenting insulin secretion and therefore are useless in severe type I diabetes. There are many sulphonylureas available but the newer ones do not seem to have any clear advantages.

Tolbutamide is relatively short-acting. The starting dose is 250 mg twice a day.

Chlorpropamide is long-acting. The dose is 100 mg each morning rising to a maximum of 500 mg.

Others include glibenclamide, glipizide, glymidine, acetohexamide, glibornuride and tolazamide. They may produce hypoglycaemia, particularly the long-acting ones in elderly patients, for whom tolbutamide is therefore preferred. The drugs are contra-indicated in ketosis and should be avoided in pregnancy. Adverse reactions are uncommon but gastro-intestinal upset and headache may occur.

Some individuals have an inherited tendency to alcohol-induced flushing when taking sulphonylureas, particularly chlorpropamide. Tolbutamide is preferred in renal failure and chlorpropamide in hepatic failure. Because of incompatibilities, hypoglycaemia may occur with the simultaneous administration of sulphonamides, salicylates, phenylbutazone, monoamine oxidase inhibitors, β-adrenergic blocking drugs and alcohol.

The majority of late-onset diabetics respond to sulphonylureas but as each year passes a small proportion of patients will escape from control. Changing to another sulphonylurea is rarely helpful and most of these 'secondary failures' will need insulin.

Biguanides

These are now going out of use because of the danger of lactic acidosis, particularly with phenformin. There may still be a place for using metformin in obese diabetics who show only a partial response to sulphonylureas.

INSULIN

This is the mainstay of treatment in severe or ketotic diabetes. Insulin is digested in the gastro-intestinal tract and all forms of insulin must be injected. Commercial insulin is all 'beef' or 'pork' at present but 'human' insulin is expected shortly. Insulin solutions or suspensions are in acetate or phosphate buffer with a little phenol or similar material as a preservative. Insulin need not be refrigerated in the UK.

Insulin is standardised by bioassay, so dosage is in units It is intended in future that all insulin will be supplied in a strength of 100 units/ml but the old strengths of 20, 40 and 80 units/ml will be available for a time.

Types of insulin

There is now a bewildering variety of insulins available and as they are not necessarily of equivalent potency for the individual great care is needed in prescribing. It is best to use a few familiar preparations. There is no need to use the acidic soluble insulin preparations and all should be at neutral pH. The older preparations, still widely used, are relatively impure and certain other proteins including proinsulin, 'C' peptide and pancreatic polypeptide. New preparations have been purified to a greater or lesser extent. It is still not clear whether they represent an advance in treatment or not but as they have long-term theoretical advantages it is usual practice to prescribe them for the newly diagnosed diabetic, particularly if young.

Many attempts have been made to produce modifications of insulin to prolong the effect of a single injection. The standard preparations are:

1. Neutral *soluble* insulin—short action
2. *Isophane* insulin—intermediate action
3. Insulin *zinc suspension* (mixed)—long action—(see Fig. 4.1)

Isophane insulin is also called 'N.P.H.' (Neutral protamine Hagedorn). Insulin zinc suspension (mixed) contains 70% of a crystalline form which is longer acting and 30% of an amorphous form which is shorter acting. Other long-acting insulins and mixtures are available. All soluble insulins are clear solutions and all longer acting ones are cloudy. Most but not all types of insulin can be mixed in the syringe.

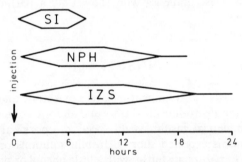

FIG. 4.1. Approximate times of onset, full effect and total duration of action after subcutaneous injection of soluble insulin (S1), isophane insulin (NPH) and insulin zinc suspension (IZS).

Technique of injection

Whenever possible patients should be taught to give their own injections. There are standard metal and glass insulin syringes, in future graduated in 100 units/ml; the syringe and needle should be kept in *methylated* spirit. Portable containers are available. Syringes should be replaced regularly or at the first sign of leakage anywhere. Disposable syringes with needles are available. The cap of the insulin bottle should be cleaned with spirit but the skin need not be cleaned. Current technique is to insert the needle at right angles to the skin and make the injection subcutaneously. Any site may be used, preferably in rotation, but the upper outer arms, front or outer thighs or abdominal wall are preferred. Careful training of the patient in injection technique is an important part of management. Various devices are available to help including guns and syringes with a fixed capacity or clicks for the partially sighted.

There is interest in the use of different systems of delivery for insulin. Intravenous infusion is well established for short-term use but in addition long-term continuous subcutaneous injection from portable pumps is being attempted.

STARTING TREATMENT WITH INSULIN

There is no standard dose of insulin; the individual's needs have to be found by trial and error.

The regime will depend on circumstances.

1. In the *late-onset diabetic*, it is likely that treatment with diet and tablets will have failed. Such patients may be started on insulin zinc suspension (IZS) (mixed) with the expectation of achieving reasonable control. Admission to hospital is not obligatory but if it is to be avoided, careful education is essential and home supervision desirable.

A diet prescription of 100 to 200 g CHO per day should be given, with a preponderance of intake at supper time.

The insulin injection should be given about half an hour before breakfast, but this is not critical. A starting dose of about 12 units of IZS is appropriate and this is increased as necessary every 2–3 days but not more quickly as there is some cumulative effect. The aim is to get the urine free from ketones and largely free from sugar at all times. When this is achieved it is useful to check plasma glucose levels two hours after meals to ensure that the urine test is a reliable guide.

If control is poor at certain times of day, it may be improved by reducing the load of carbohydrate at those times or by adding additional amounts of amorphous (quick acting, 'Semilente') or crystalline (long-acting, 'Ultralente') IZS to the prescription but this latter complication is best avoided. Neutral soluble insulin may be added also. If total requirements are over about 40 units a day, IZS is unlikely to be satisfactory and two injections of soluble insulin or soluble-plus-isophane insulin may be better.

2. In the *younger patient* with greater ketosis, in severe intercurrent illness or after an episode of ketoacidosis, for example, a different approach is needed. Control may be established using soluble insulin and a permanent regime selected later. A diet should be prescribed as soon as possible. At first, soluble insulin should be injected before each main meal, or eight hourly if the patient is on an intravenous regime. A

suitable starting dose might be 8 or 12 units each time, increasing rapidly as necessary. Much larger amounts and frequent changes of dose may be needed. A 'sliding scale' of insulin in which the dose is predetermined in relation to the plasma glucose may be used. For good care at this difficult stage of treatment there is no alternative to close supervision and frequent adjustment of insulin dose.

When reasonable control has been established or immediately in the milder case a decision has to be made about the pattern of long-term treatment. The diet prescription should be adjusted to take account of the patient's usual routine. For nearly all Type I diabetics a twice daily injection is needed. Opinions differ as to the best combination but the author prefers Isophane and soluble insulin. A total daily requirement of 48 units of insulin might be deployed as:

7.00 a.m.   Isophane— 16 units ⎫ mixed
            Neutral soluble— 12 units ⎬
6.00 p.m.   Isophane— 12 units ⎫ mixed
            Neutral soluble— 8 units ⎬

This would assume a medium sized breakfast, large lunch and moderate supper with a late evening snack.

After 48 h the schedule is adjusted depending on glycosuria or plasma glucose levels. For example—high plasma glucose before lunch: increase morning isophane; evening hypoglycaemia: reduce evening soluble. It is not useful to achieve meticulous control in hospital because after discharge the change in diet and exercise will alter insulin requirements and further adjustments will be needed.

Alternative regimes use insulin zinc suspension, mixed with short-acting forms, and soluble insulin alone, two or three times a day. Isophane alone is not likely to be satisfactory but is sometimes effective if given twice a day. There are innumerable different regimes of insulin treatment and the only criterion is success for the individual patient—if control is satisfactory there is no reason to change.

Difficulties during treatment

Unless mentally or physically handicapped, insulin-dependent diabetics should be encouraged to adjust their own dose of insulin when necessary. Generally, doses should not be changed more frequently than every 2 days and by no more than 4 units at a time. The best time to test the blood or urine varies with the regime, but it is generally better to check before meals. In the well controlled diabetic urine testing once a week will suffice but it should be done several times on the same day.

Physical exertion reduces insulin requirements so return to hard physical work will need a reduction of dose by as much as 20%. Problems arise particularly with intercurrent illness which, even if mild, increases insulin needs. Nausea or vomiting may cause difficulty. It is important that the diabetic does not omit the insulin because no food has been taken—indeed, an increased dose may be appropriate. Failure to observe this rule may lead to ketoacidosis. Variable shift working should be discouraged but is possible if the treatment is adjusted with care.

Successful control of the diabetes may cause alteration in vision as the refractive power of the lens changes with the plasma glucose; new spectacles may be needed.

Is strict diabetic control worthwhile?

For the younger diabetic particularly this question is crucial but not easy to answer. Presumably a well-controlled diabetic is at less risk of unexpected ketoacidosis and hypoglycaemia. There is some evidence that good control reverses or slows the progress of complications such as retinopathy and neuropathy. However, it has never been *proved* that good control prevents or delays complications and indeed most diabetics develop complications eventually, however good their control. It seems rational to suppose that the raised plasma glucose has something to do with the complications and therefore careful control is recommended and encouraged but it must be admitted that proof of benefit is elusive.

Adverse reactions to insulin

Local

If the injection is placed in the subcutaneous tissues there is usually no problem, but correct technique is important. It may be helpful to observe the patient giving the injection. If the injection is made into the skin it is more painful and causes skin damage. About two weeks after starting insulin a local reaction may develop for 1–2 cm around the injection sites and last several days. This reaction diminishes after a few weeks if the same treatment is continued or alternatively a different form of insulin may be used. Repeated injections at one site may produce a fibro-fatty mass. This is unsightly and insulin injected into it may be absorbed unevenly. The remedy is to inject elsewhere into numerous different sites.

General

A generalised sensitivity reaction may follow the injection of insulin, just as after any other protein, but is very rare. Treatment is with adrenaline and corticosteroids. Desensitisation may be required.

Hypoglycaemia

Despite its great benefits insulin treatment is dangerous because of the risk of hypoglycaemia. This is most likely to occur at the peaks of insulin effect and will vary with the type of insulin. Long-acting insulin producing hypoglycaemia during sleep is a particular hazard. Hypoglycaemia is most commonly caused by a missed or inadequate meal but an inadvertent (or even deliberate) overdose of insulin has the same effect, as may severe or prolonged exercise. Hypoglycaemia may be troublesome soon after initiation of insulin treatment due to falling insulin requirement with good control, or an increase in physical activity after return to work. Sometimes hypoglycaemia occurs for no apparent reason.

The symptoms are quite variable and those from long-acting insulins may be atypical. Acute falls in plasma glucose are likely to produce sweating, palpitations and hunger while slower changes tend to lead to unusual or irrational behaviour going on to unsteadiness, tremor, diplopia, paraesthesiae, drowsiness and coma, sometimes within a few minutes.

The diagnosis is suspected if the patient is known to be on insulin, has subcutaneous injection marks or carries identification as a diabetic. The skin is pale, the pulse and respiration are normal and there is no dehydration. An epileptic fit may occur, and following it the signs may be complicated by post-ictic changes. Urine tests are unreliable as the bladder may hold urine secreted earlier and containing sugar. A plasma glucose estimation (below 2.5 mmol/l) is diagnostic. If in doubt, give glucose.

Treatment

Every patient starting on insulin must learn about hypoglycaemia. Hypoglycaemia should be induced in every new diabetic so that they know what it feels like. A diabetic on insulin should always carry at least 30 g of sugar (e.g. boiled sweets) and use it to abort hypoglycaemia. It is necessary to treat a patient with hypoglycaemia with 20 g of carbohydrate. Glucose or sugar by mouth should be given at once if possible and repeated every few minutes as necessary. If the patient cannot swallow, 20 ml of a 50% solution of glucose should be given intravenously. Glucose down a nasogastric tube is a slower alternative. Both should be followed by carbohydrate food as soon as consciousness returns. It is important to appreciate that there is no fixed dose of sugar in treating hypoglycaemia but as much as is necessary to control symptoms must be given. An alternative is to give glucagon 1 mg subcutaneously. Rarely, consciousness does not return quickly. If so, the diagnosis must be reconsidered—if no other cause for the coma can be found the plasma glucose is maintained in the hope of later recovery, which may be after many days. If in doubt about the diagnosis always take blood for glucose measurement *before* treatment.

N.B. All diabetics on insulin carry a card at all times identifying them as being diabetic and showing their treatment regime.

SELECTION OF TREATMENT

The following suggestions will cover most eventualities.
1. If the diabetes is mild and the patient is asymptomatic, particularly in the elderly, only minor dietary advice is needed.
2. If the patient is frankly diabetic but asymptomatic, treatment is justified in the hope of retarding complications.
3. If the patient is obese, weight reduction should be attempted.
4. If the patient has no ketosis, dietary treatment alone should be tried first.
5. If diet fails and there is no ketosis, add sulphonylureas.
6. If the patient is young and has ketosis, insulin will be needed.
7. If there is marked or persistent ketosis, or if marked hyperglycaemia is resistant to treatment, insulin will be needed.
8. Do not press treatment with unnecessary vigour, particularly in the elderly.

SUPERVISION

Only the patients can supervise their own treatment continuously and this should be encouraged whenever possible. For the doctor, nurse or health visitor, called upon to advise occasionally, the decision to intervene or not can be difficult. Despite the uncertainties in defining a philosophy of management, the following four basic situations provide useful guidelines:
1. If the patient denies symptoms, has no more than occasional glycosuria, and the post-prandial plasma glucose is < 10 mmol/l, this degree of control is acceptable. Occasional higher levels of plasma glucose are acceptable also, particularly in the elderly or if there is a transient cause such as an infection or celebration.

2. If symptoms such as polydipsia and pruritus persist there must be significant glycosuria, whatever the tests are alleged to show, and stricter treatment should be advised.
3. If the post-prandial plasma glucose is persistently > 15 mmol/l treatment should be adjusted.
4. If there is significant ketosis (usually with a plasma glucose > 20 mmol/l) better control is urgently necessary.

There are nevertheless innumerable individual variations calling for individual decisions. The measurement of glycosylated haemoglobin as a measure of long-term diabetic control is being evaluated.

SPECIAL CIRCUMSTANCES

Children

The treatment of diabetic children follows the general pattern of that for adults. The diabetes is usually insulin-dependent and after initial treatment with doses of soluble insulin appropriate for size and severity, twice daily injections as for adults are preferred. Free diets have been used but rarely give reasonable control and a carbohydrate controlled diet is indicated. The diet should be generous to encourage normal development although usually growth and maturity are some-what delayed. Emotional problems are to be expected in such a difficult situation and much will depend on the parents for whom long-term advice and support may be vital.

'Brittle' diabetes

This term is applied to those few diabetics in whom insulin requirements fluctuate widely for no apparent reason The cause is not clear but emotional lability or non-compliance may be relevant.

Insulin resistance

Rarely, a state of severe resistance to insulin appears, perhaps because of the development of antibodies, and insulin needs may rise to several hundred units a day. Treatment with corticosteroids may help and the condition remits after a few months.

Pregnancy

Three quite distinct circumstances need to be considered.

Glycosuria
The renal threshold for sugar tends to fall during pregnancy, particularly after the first trimester, so glycosuria is common. A plasma glucose measurement or glucose tolerance test is needed to determine whether the woman has become diabetic or not.

'Gestational diabetes'
This term is applied to those women who become diabetic and require treatment during pregnancy but whose glucose tolerance returns to normal after delivery.

Pregnancy in established diabetes
Because of the age group most pregnant diabetics are insulin-dependent but occasionally diet alone will suffice. Sulphonylureas should be avoided. During pregnancy insulin requirements rise from the fourth month and the tendency to a lower renal glucose threshold means that reliance must be placed on plasma glucose measurements. With reasonable care, the risk to the mother is negligible but the risk of fetal or neonatal death is still higher than in non-diabetics, even with good control.

There is an increased risk of toxaemia, hydramnios and placental infarcts, and the fetus tends to be large. Treatment is by meticulous control of the diabetes throughout the pregnancy, with frequent review of the diabetic and obstetric situation. The prevention of ketoacidosis is particularly important. Insulin dose is increased as necessary and the diet controlled to ensure optimum weight. Swift admission to hospital, repeatedly if necessary, is indicated if more than trivial problems arise, and also in the later weeks.

During the final stages of pregnancy careful fetal monitoring is necessary with early induction of labour if fetal distress occurs. If labour does not begin, induction between the 36th–38th week is usually recommended.

During labour, plasma glucose is controlled by injections of soluble insulin every 6–8 h with i.v. glucose. Insulin infusion may be used (see ketoacidosis, below). After delivery, insulin requirement falls suddenly and it is given according to need. The baby tends to be large and is liable to various complications so requires careful supervision. Hypoglycaemia may need treatment.

Menstruation

Many women notice a change in their insulin requirements during the menstrual cycle with a tendency towards increased insulin needs during the menses but the changes are not consistent. Each woman needs to observe her own pattern and adjust her treatment accordingly.

Family planning

With current therapy the risk to life of pregnancy for a diabetic is minimal but there are other considerations and family planning is particularly important for the diabetic. The miscarriage rate is still quite high and the risk of congenital malformations is increased. Also, there is a small but distinct risk of the child becoming diabetic. More important, pregnancy may accelerate diabetic complications. A diabetic should consider her own health and possible future disability in relation to the welfare of her family. It is perhaps best that a diabetic who wishes to have children (preferably only two) should do so quickly and early. Thereafter sterilisation should be offered but as it is the woman's health which is particularly at risk it is best to recommend tubal ligation rather than vasectomy. Alternatively, the safest course of action is probably barrier methods coupled with termination of pregnancy in the event of failure. If this is unacceptable, then both the intrauterine contraceptive device and the combined oral contraceptive may be used. In both cases there may be a slightly greater risk than for the non-diabetic but published reports are conflicting. The place of the progestogen only pill is uncertain. The choice of oral contraceptive preparation can be made on general grounds (see Chapter 13). When it is begun there may be a small increase in insulin needs but thereafter control is as good or bad as before. Review every six months is important: if major diabetic complications appear the oral contraceptive should be stopped. Pregnancy is then contra-indicated also and sometimes termination of pregnancy may have to be recommended.

Surgery

Treatment should be reviewed before any major surgical procedure. If the diabetes is controlled by diet and/or tablets it is sufficient to continue treatment until the night before and then omit food and tablets on the day of operation. The urine must be tested regularly and treatment is resumed as soon as possible. If glycosuria appears, particularly with ketosis, as may well happen after a major operation, plasma glucose should be estimated and if necessary controlled temporarily with soluble insulin. Ketosis without a raised plasma glucose will be due to starvation and does not require treatment. If the patient is on insulin it is usually prudent to change to soluble insulin injected two or three times daily for two or three days. This period should be extended if necessary until reasonable control is obtained. On the day of operation half the usual morning dose of soluble insulin is given with a slow infusion of 5% dextrose i.v. For emergency surgery these arrangements may be impossible and then soluble insulin is given as necessary to control the plasma glucose. The glucose infusion should be continued until the patient can take food, and insulin dosage is reviewed twice a day depending on plasma glucose. Alternatively, intravenous or subcutaneous insulin infusions may be used. Hypoglycaemia is the greater risk. As soon as possible the patient's usual routine is restored.

Other treatment

The treatment of intercurrent illness in diabetics may need special care. Diuretics may reduce carbohydrate tolerance but frusemide seems satisfactory. Corticosteroids antagonise the action of insulin and their systemic use should be restricted. The sugar content of coated tablets is too small to be important but syrups should be avoided. Some drugs potentiate the actions of sulphonylureas (see above) and cause hypoglycaemia. β-adrenergic blocking drugs can be used but mask some features of hypoglycaemia and retard recovery from it; the selective β_1-blockers such as atenolol and acebutolol are safer in this respect.

THE TREATMENT OF DIABETIC COMPLICATIONS

Ketoacidosis

This is an emergency and calls for urgent treatment. The essentials are intravenous saline and insulin. If the patient is drowsy or unconscious admission to hospital is necessary.

Saline

On arrival, an intravenous infusion of 0.9% saline is started at a rate of 1–2 1/h (adults). Venous blood is taken for measurement of glucose and electrolytes, including bicarbonate. If possible, blood gases and pH should be estimated. The stomach should be aspirated if the patient is unconscious or if gastric dilatation is suspected.

Insulin

Small, frequent doses of insulin are an effective emergency treatment—various regimes may be used.

1. Continuous i.v. infusion of soluble insulin from a syringe pump at the rate of about 5 units/h. Fresh insulin solutions should be prepared every six hours. Mixing insulin in an infusion bottle is less satisfactory because of loss of insulin on to the glass or plastic surfaces.
2. Soluble insulin i.m. initially of 10 units then 5 units each hour.

Bicarbonate
This need not be given routinely but if the blood pH is below 7.1, 100 mmol of sodium bicarbonate may be given over 2 h (e.g. 250 ml of 3% sodium bicarbonate). More bicarbonate may be given later if severe acidosis persists.

Potassium
This should not be given until the plasma potassium level is known. If normal or low, potassium chloride at a rate of 10–20 mmol (0.75–1.5 gm) is given *slowly* intravenously during each hour.

N.B. Both i.v. bicarbonate and potassium are dangerous treatments and must be controlled with care—slow administration is essential.

Any precipitating cause for the ketoacidosis (e.g. infection) should be sought and treated.

Progress
Careful observation with a plasma glucose measurement every two hours is desirable. Any urine passed should be tested for ketones. The fluid transfusion rate should be slowed when there is a good urine output and blood pressure, or if signs of cardiac failure appear. With insulin infusion a steady fall of glucose may be expected and the time of reaching normality predicted.

When the plasma glucose reaches 10–20 mmol/l the transfusion fluid is changed to dextrose saline and the insulin regime changed to subcutaneous injections of soluble insulin every six or eight hours as needed, perhaps for a further 24 h. As soon as possible, a regular regime of diet and insulin is established.

Non-ketotic hyperosmolar diabetes
A similar regime is used except that half normal saline is given.

'Diabetic feet'
Atheroma. Gangrene due to major arterial obstruction will require amputation at the lowest level possible to achieve a viable stump.

Peripheral arterial obstruction. With a reasonably good major arterial supply, gangrene can sometimes be treated successfully by a limited resection of the toe(s) or part of the foot.

Neuropathic blisters and ulcers are treated by elevation of the foot for much of the day and relief of pressure on the lesion.

Sepsis. This often complicates the lesions mentioned above; it requires systemic antibiotics to control surrounding cellulitis with local cleansing and dressings.

Microvascular

Retinopathy
Minor changes do not call for local treatment. It is usual to recommend strict diabetic control and this may be of value in slowing progression of the lesions, but does not help in all patients. Light coagulation of areas of the retina has been shown to be a useful treatment. It destroys blood vessels, relieves oedema and inhibits new vessel formation. The xenon arc produces white light and this causes maximum damage at the pigment epithelium with destruction of overlying vessels. The argon laser is probably better as it produces a much narrower light beam (50 μm or less) and can therefore be used near the macula. Its colour (green) leads to maximum energy absorption by haemoglobin and therefore the vessels are damaged primarily. Light coagulation is indicated if there is new vessel formation on the disc or retina, or maculopathy. Retinopathy must be detected early so that treatment may be considered.

Nephropathy
There is no specific treatment. Low protein diet regimes for progressive renal failure may be indicated, as well as treatment for hypertension. Renal dialysis and transplantation are difficult because of the high incidence of complications but may become possible with better techniques.

Neuropathy
There is no specific treatment. It is usual to give vitamin B complex but there is no evidence that it is of value and it is used as a harmless and cheap placebo. For painful neuropathy pain relief techniques may be needed. Sometimes anticonvulsants such as phenytoin, carbamazepine and sodium valproate are helpful.

Atheroma

The general treatment of occlusion of major arteries in diabetes (e.g. myocardial infarction or stroke) does not differ from that in the non-diabetic.

EDUCATION

The education of the diabetic is an essential and continuing feature of management and good diabetic control is unlikely unless the diabetic understands and cooperates in treatment. Particular points are:

Literature
There is an extensive literature for patients available from many sources including the British Diabetic Association (see Further Reading) and there may be meetings of local branches of the Association which the diabetic can attend. Supervision by doctors and nurses should include attempts to find out if the patient understands the problems and also time for questions and answers.

Instruction and demonstration
Is needed to teach the techniques of insulin administration, care of equipment, urine testing and blood testing.

Diet
A diet sheet should be provided.

Feet
Hygiene.

Control of treatment
Most insulin dependent diabetics can learn to carry out considerable manipulation of their treatment with changes of insulin dose and diet when required and this is to be encouraged.

ORGANISATION

In-patients

Because of the nature of the disease some special arrangements are desirable during in-patient care. A stock of appropriate literature should be available. An appropriate diet must be provided—if this is not possible, let the patients select their own food from what is available and bring in what else is required. Normal ward routine may need to be modified to ensure insulin injections at the correct times. A 'diabetic chart' is essential. This includes recording of quantitative urine analysis for glucose and ketones every six hours, plasma glucose when measured and all insulin injections. The presence of nurses experienced in diabetes is invaluable.

Diabetic out-patient clinics

The role of these clinics is changing with more emphasis on education. There is a welcome trend towards greater involvement of family practitioners in the treatment of diabetes. The clinic is useful for establishing the diagnosis, initiating treatment and beginning the patient's education. A review, including retinoscopy, at one or two yearly intervals by a doctor is useful but it does not have to be done at a hospital. The presence of a dietitian, chiropodist and laboratory services means that the clinic attendance can be a comprehensive review. Of course, the value of occasional plasma glucose measurements is of questionable value because some patients only take their diabetes seriously when a clinic attendance is due, but that is better than nothing and reinforces the need for supervision somewhere. For older or infirm patients the community nursing service may have to undertake the insulin injections and day to day supervision.

THE DIABETIC LIFE

Diabetics, particularly if on insulin, have long-term risks of complications but there must always be a determined effort by them and their advisers to ensure that the proper management of their diabetes causes minimal interference with normal life. This attitude, which is supported strongly by membership of the British Diabetic Association is sensible not only in general terms but also in encouraging the cooperation of the patients; the diabetic should look forward to a full and useful life.

FURTHER READING

ALBERTI K.G.M.M. & THOMAS D.J.B. (1979). The management of diabetes during surgery. *British Journal of Anaesthesia*, **51**, 693.
BLOOM A. (1978). *Diabetes Explained* (3rd Edition) MTP Press, Lancaster.

BRITISH DIABETIC ASSOCIATION, Various publications. 10, Queen Anne Street, London W1M 0BD (Tel 01–323 1531).

ESSEX N. (1976). Diabetes and pregnancy. *British Journal of Hospital Medicine*, **15**, 333.

HILL R.D. (1976). Running a diabetic clinic. *British Journal of Hospital Medicine*, **16**, 218.

KEEN H. & JARRETT J. (Eds.) (1975). *Complications of diabetes* Edward Arnold, London.

OAKLEY W.G. *et al* (1978). *Diabetes and its Management* (3rd Edition) Blackwell Scientific Publications, Oxford.

Chapter 5
Obesity

CONSEQUENCES OF OBESITY

Obese people are likely to die younger than thin people but the difference is great only with severe obesity (see definition below). Some of the ill effects are indirect and mediated by the association of obesity with hypertension, diabetes and raised blood lipids. There is increased morbidity in the obese because of loss of mobility, osteoarthritis, gall stones and complications of parturition and surgery.

49

The psychological and social consequences are important also with obvious difficulties in social contacts, employment, holidays and clothes. In current Western culture, with its emphasis on appearances and publicity for slimness, the burden of even moderate obesity can be hard to bear. Amongst young women a substantial proportion are trying to lose weight at any one time and over a year probably a majority have tried to do so.

DEFINITION

A precise definition of obesity is elusive. Presumably it would be ideal to measure total body fat and compare with tables of normality. Body fat can be measured with moderate accuracy with skin fold calipers but the method is less reliable in the very obese. Accurate methods are complex and not suitable for routine use. Satisfactory 'normal' values are not available.

An alternative is to use an 'obesity index' such as body weight (kg)/height^2 (m). The normal range for this index is 20–25 (male) and 19–24 (female).

In practice it is usual to use the patient's body weight and taking account of age and sex, compare it with a chart of 'ideal' weight (Fig. 5.1), that is to say the weight associated with greatest longevity. No allowance is made for age but there is an allowance for frame size and this poses a problem. A person with heavy bone structure and musculature has a higher 'ideal' weight than a person with a small frame. There is no standard method of assessing frame size and the chart shows values which were graded according to the impression of the observers. To use the chart you have to do the same. It is best to consider the skeleton and note the width of the wrist and shoulders, and the size of the head, as these dimensions are little effected by the degree of obesity. In doubt, use the 'medium frame' values. The patient's weight can be expressed as a percentage of the mean for the appropriate frame size. Up to 110% is considered to be within the normal range, 110–130% as obese and over 130% severely obese.

PREVALENCE

The prevalence of obesity varies in different societies at different times. In the UK nearly half of all adults between 30 and 50 years of age are more than 10% overweight with nearly one in five being more than

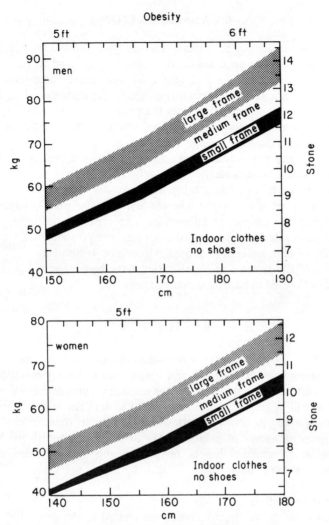

FIG. 5.1. The range of desirable weight for height in people over 25. Weight in indoor clothes, height in stockinged feet. The judgement of frame size is subjective. Reprinted by permission of Medical Education (International) Ltd.

20% overweight. In post-menopausal women about a third are more than 20% overweight whereas men of the same age are less effected. The reason for the sex difference is not clear. At their ideal weights a woman has about 20% of her weight in fat whereas a man has only 10% but whether this predisposes to excessive fat in women is not known. Common observation suggests considerable social class and ethnic differences but these are poorly documented.

CLASSIFICATION

There have been many attempts to classify types of obesity. The distribution of fat has been considered—some women tend to have large deposits on the buttocks and thighs whereas most obese men have relatively thin legs with excess fat on and in the abdomen. It is likely that these distributions reflect only the proportions of the fat deposits in different individuals irrespective of whether they are fat or thin. Changes in fat deposits are approximately proportional—if a fat layer doubles at one site it doubles at another. Obesity accentuates the fat pattern but does not cause it.

'Hypertrophic' obesity is taken to mean an increase in *size* of a normal number of adipocytes whereas 'hyperplastic' obesity implies an increase in the *number* of adipocytes. Experimental confirmation of this concept is lacking. The age of onset has been considered, i.e. before or after puberty, again in relationship to adipocyte numbers.

None of the systems of classification have been accepted generally nor have they led to improved management.

AETIOLOGY

In nutrition, physical energy is measured in terms of heat; this applies to the energy content of food and tissues and to energy metabolism. The SI unit of heat is the joule but the traditional unit of the *kilocalorie* (kcal) is still in general use (1 kcal = 4.2 kjoule). The laws of thermodynamics apply in obesity as elsewhere; excess fat deposits can arise only from an excess of calorie intake above consumption so that a discussion of aetiology has to revolve around the two sides of the equation of energy balance.

Appetite and satiety
Certain areas of the hypothalamus are related to the *desire* for food. Rarely hypothalamic disease may increase appetite and the effect of drugs (e.g. cyproheptadine) in this direction may be mediated through these centres. Many illnesses such as hepatitis and non-specific changes such as fever suppress appetite but the mechanism is unknown. It is proposed that other hypothalamic centres control *satiety*, i.e. the sensation when appetite has been assuaged but the practical significance of this concept is uncertain.

Metabolism
The digestion and absorbtion of nutrients is the same in the obese as in

others and the excretion of calories in the urine and faeces is the same also.

There is a normal adaptation which changes the rate of metabolism to some extent in response to calorie intake—increased food increases metabolism and reduced food reduces it. There is evidence that this system is modified in the obese so that there is a subnormal increase in metabolism with extra food but an enhanced response to food restriction. Consequently the obese person tends to retain calories when overeating but conserves calories well when food is restricted. The magnitude and significance of this change in obesity is uncertain but presumably it has survival value when food supply fluctuates as it implies a greater than normal efficiency in energy conservation.

A possible biochemical mediation for this system is the deiodination of T_4. If it leads to 'ordinary' T_3, which is highly potent, calorie expenditure would be increased whereas if the process deviated towards the production of 'reverse' T_3, which is inert, calorie conservation might result.

Exercise
Physical exercise uses calories and in this respect obese persons are relatively inefficient because their bulk increases the energy cost of physical activity. It has been postulated that obese persons are relatively physically inactive but the evidence is conflicting. In industrialised societies, energy expenditure through physical work is relatively low. Individuals such as housewives who correctly consider themselves to be busy and who work long hours, nevertheless expend relatively few calories. Exercise has to be very strenuous, e.g. cross-country running, before calorie expenditure rises much above 500 kcal/h.

Adipose tissue cells
Ordinary adipocytes in the obese do not appear to have any metabolic defect and can synthesise, take up and release lipid in the normal way. There are specialised adipose tissue cells in *brown adipose tissue* (BAT or 'brown fat'). Brown fat occurs in small localised deposits, e.g. beneath the skin between the shoulder blades. BAT cells have a low fat content but are metabolically active and liberate heat. Whether they are important in calorie adaptation in man remains to be seen— the total mass of BAT may be too small to be of importance.

Social and genetic factors
Obese persons tend to have obese parents and vice versa. This could be genetic or environmental through the eating habits inculcated in the

child by the family. Feminists have proposed that the higher incidence of obesity in women is related to their role in contemporary society.

Other aspects of society may be important also. The preparation, giving and taking of food have important social implications in the structure of family life and social intercourse. There is a great variety of food available at prices nearly all can afford. There is a trend towards the use of processed foods with relatively high fat and refined carbohydrate contents and little fibre. Such foods are concentrated sources of calories and many can be eaten as snacks at any time of day. Alcoholic beverages are consumed in large and increasing quantities so that they now provide over 5% of total calorie intake in the UK.

Overeating

It is popularly believed (particularly by the slim) that obesity is due to gluttony and in some obese persons this is so. Also, some obese people report intermittent eating 'binges' with weight gain. However, common observation suggests that large eaters may be slim and studies with careful dietary histories now indicate that on average the obese have about the same calorie intake as the slim. Even so, dietary histories are notoriously unreliable and a small consistent calorie excess will in time cause major weight gain.

Type of food

Although it is a common belief that the type of food eaten contributes to obesity, this is not certain. A diet high in concentrated foods may actually have less power to relieve hunger and so encourage overeating. High fibre foods are bulky and perhaps more satisfying; also, fibre retards intestinal absorption. Starchy foods in themselves cannot be blamed.

The digestion, absorption and assimilation of food has its own energy cost; this has been called 'specific dynamic action' and the more modern term 'dietary induced thermogenesis' refers to the same process. It might be that different foods prepared or taken in different ways have variable effects and this might be important in energy balance but little information is available.

Salt and water content of the diet are not relevant. Carbohydrate intake affects sodium balance through unknown mediators. However, the changes in body sodium occur only within the normal range so that the effect on weight is small. There is no effect on body fat but the changes in body weight through fluid retention may be of psychological importance during attempts at slimming (see below).

Diagnosis

Few patients presenting for advice about obesity have any detectable endocrinological disorder, but it is important to be alert to the possibility, particularly as many patients believe that they have a glandular fault and may benefit from specific reassurance as part of their management. There are three endocrine conditions related to obesity which should be considered routinely.

Hypothyroidism
It is unusual for this to be associated with gross obesity. The history should help—if the obesity is of long standing and not associated with general symptoms or specific complaints such as constipation or cold intolerance etc., then hypothyroidism is unlikely. Physical examination should reveal the gross case, but the measurement of plasma thyroxine is a cheap and efficient screening test which should be used freely if in doubt.

Polycystic ovary syndrome
Obesity associated with irregular periods and hirsutism will suggest this diagnosis (see Chapter 12).

Cushing's syndrome
The physical examination is more likely to be of value than the history (unless corticosteroid drugs have been given) and it is important to seek striae and hypertension (see Chapter 9). The differentiation between the common simple obesity with rapid weight gain (which may cause striae) and the rare Cushing's syndrome, may be difficult— isolated measurements of plasma cortisol in outpatients are of limited value but an overnight dexamethasone supression test is simple and moderately reliable.

A general medical history and physical examination is important to identify any other problem, e.g. arthritis, which may affect management.

MANAGEMENT

The diagnosis of simple obesity and its degree having been made, an early decision about the *style* of management is needed. This needs to be tailored to the needs of the individual; in the elderly moderately overweight female, for example, vigorous treatment would not be appropriate because of its difficulty and dubious benefit, but there may be special circumstances such as diabetes or the need for surgery.

If a determined effort at slimming is to be made, then a careful interview is needed to establish rapport and explore the individual's circumstances. The discussion should include:

1. The history of the patient's weight and the family history.
2. Patient's job, including degree of physical exertion and role in food preparation.
3. Eating habits.
4. Understanding of nutrition and attitude towards food and dieting.
5. Motivation—internal or external attitude of relatives.
6. Financial resources.

Exposition

A sympathetic attitude is essential but it is necessary to emphasise tive should be for the patient to change his/her habits permanently so makes no difference what I eat' (as many do) are likely to be hostile to advice and present a formidable challenge. The long-term objective should be for the patient to change their habits permanently so that not only will weight be lost, but that the benefit be maintained. It may be helpful to set a target weight but this needs discretion—an unreasonable target may reduce motivation. It is rarely profitable to cover all these matters at the first interview.

Diet

A relative reduction in calorie intake is a prerequisite for weight reduction so some advice about diet is essential. The innumerable types of diet which have been recommended is good evidence that none is generally advantageous.

Calorie content
A target of about 2500 kcal/d would be suitable for a man doing physical work whereas for a short, relatively inactive woman 1000 kcal/d would be appropriate. More restrictive diets are unlikely to be acceptable and extreme diets or total starvation are not recommended because they are hazardous.

'What should I eat?'
There is no good evidence that the nature of the food has any long-term

effect on weight, but it is difficult to convince the patient of this. One of the most pernicious popular misconceptions is that different foods are more or less 'fattening'. Also, some people believe, partly due to advertising, that some foods are *positively* helpful and that their consumption will lead to weight loss. It is unfortunate that foods widely regarded as 'fattening' such as bread and potatoes have relatively low calorie concentrations compared, say, to meat which always contains a lot of fat (twice as many calories per gram as carbohydrate) and therefore a concentrated source of calories. The foods generally thought desirable such as meat, fruit and salads tend to be expensive, sometimes difficult to get and may be little to the patient's taste.

The patient's normal eating habits should be respected as far as possible. It is usual to recommend three small meals a day, but some people manage with two. An effective weight reducing diet can be constructed entirely from the foods which the patient normally eats provided that the quantities are appropriate. Such advice has the advantage of practicality and cost. Some patients respond well to advice about what foods to avoid and providing they are frugal about quantities of permitted food, a good result will follow. There is no need to restrict water intake nor to recommend any special (and usually expensive) low calorie foods. There is a theoretical risk of nutritional deficiencies from a low calorie diet but in practice this must be extremely rare.

Some written guidelines are most helpful and are available commercially or from hospital dietetic departments. The services of a dietitian are invaluable and should be sought if possible. For the more literate patient, the book *Which? Way to Slim* (see Further reading) can be recommended.

Exercise

The calorie needs of exercise are relatively low so that considering the restriction imposed by time available, facilities, aptitude and mobility, most patients can gain little benefit. Nevertheless, any exercise is on the helpful side of the energy equation so slimmers should be urged to increase their exercise as far as possible.

Problems during treatment

This is one of the most important aspects of management. Most slimmers run into difficulties and it is helpful if they are warned in advance and understand the problems.

When a low calorie diet is instituted, weight loss is rapid at first, particularly in the very obese, as excess water is lost. This may raise unreasonable expectations and disappointment when weight loss slows down after a few weeks as water loss is completed. Even on a strict diet the loss of a kilogram of *fat* a week is as much as can be expected. As bulk is lost and there is adaptation to a low calorie intake, negative calorie balance falls and, in the same diet, weight loss may be distressingly slow.

Another problem is fluctuations in weight because of variations in body water masking fat loss. Sometimes weight remains steady for days or weeks because of this effect. If the diet is maintained the water is lost eventually, sometimes abruptly. Over a few hours or days the carbohydrate content of the diet may affect sodium balance and therefore water balance through the normal physiology of anti-diuretic hormone. A sudden intake of carbohydrate leads to sodium (and water) retention and is the cause of the well known weight gain (maybe several kilograms) from a weekend's 'dietary indiscretion'. All these effects may lead the patient to conclude that the diet is useless.

Some patients become depressed when in negative calorie balance. The reason is not known but it is a common cause of default. The value of anti-depressant drugs is uncertain.

Aids to treatment

Behaviour modification
Psychological theory proposes that some obese persons have lost the normal habit of eating appropriately because of misinterpretation of signals or 'cues' which initiate or control that behaviour. Adherence to a low calorie diet may be aided if the patient can be persuaded to modify their eating behaviour, e.g. to eat only at certain times of day and at a table with cutlery.

Slimming clubs
These have been introduced widely, both commercially and by hospital departments. They have the advantage of a non-medical environment and provide time for explanation and discussion, sharing of problems and regular follow-up. Some patients find the financial and competitive incentives helpful.

Local treatment
Methods are available which are alleged to reduce fat specifically at certain sites, but their effectiveness is unproven.

DRUGS

Hormone treatments have been recommended but only thyroid hormones have any rational basis. They cannot be recommended routinely as only doses causing hyperthyroidism have any significant effect.

There are several *appetite-suppressing drugs* available which are only rarely habit forming. Their effects are short lived (4–6 weeks) and although they may be helpful at the introduction of a weight reducing diet, their overall advantage is doubtful and the author does not use them.

MECHANICAL AND SURGICAL PROCEDURES

In resistant severe obesity more extreme measures may be considered.

Jaw wiring
The teeth are fastened together by a dental splint so that only a liquid diet can be taken—this must of course be restricted in amount. Relapse after removal of the splint is usual but behavioural methods may help.

Intestinal surgery
Many operations have been devised to allow the food to bypass most of the absorbing area of the small intestine. Despite this intention, the results are due not to malabsorption but to a reduced ability to eat. The results in terms of weight loss are excellent but the morbidity and mortality rates are substantial. Plication of the stomach may be safer but equally effective.

FOLLOW-UP

With the exception of the major surgical procedures, the long-term results of weight reducing regimes of all kinds are very poor, with a success rate generally accepted as less than 5%. One of the most depressing aspects for the therapist is the high 'drop-out' rate.

CONCLUSION

We badly need better techniques to help the obese but in the meantime we can try and use the slowly increasing understanding of the metabolism and psychology of obesity. Patients can be spared useless drugs, over-complex and expensive diets, unreasonable expectations and dangerous surgery. The many alternative means of help now available can be deployed to their best advantage.

FURTHER READING

ANON (1978). *Which? Way to Slim.* Consumers Association, London.

GARROW J.S. (1978). *Energy Balance and Obesity In Man (2nd Edition).* Elsevier, Amsterdam.

GARROW J.S. (1979). Weight penalties. *British Medical Journal, ii,* 1171.

JAMES W.P.T. (Compiler) (1976). *Research on Obesity: A Report of the DHSS/MRC Group* HMSO, London.

JAMES W.P.T. & TRAYHURN P. (1981). Thermogenesis and obesity. *British Medical Bulletin,* **37** (1), 43.

MAHLER R.F. (1978). Fat: the good, the bad and the ugly. *Journal of the Royal College of Physicians,* **12,** 107.

MAXWELL J.D. *et al* (Eds) (1980). *Surgical Management in Obesity* Academic Press, London.

MUNROW J.F. *et al* (Ed) (1980). *The Treatment of Obesity* MTP Press, Lancaster.

WING R.R. & JEFFERY R.W. (1979). Out patient treatment of obesity: a comparison of methodology and clinical results. *International Journal of Obesity,* 3, 261.

Chapter 6
Thyroid

ANATOMY

The thyroid gland weighs 15–25 g and consists of two lateral lobes which are applied closely to the trachea and joined by an isthmus about 2 cm across, the upper border of which is just below the cricoid cartilage. The gland has a capsule formed by the pre-tracheal layer of the deep fascia which is attached to the cricoid cartilage and makes the gland move with the larynx during swallowing.

Histologically the gland is composed of irregular lobules each containing 20–40 follicles. A follicle or acinus averages 200 μm across. It is a sphere of 'colloid' surrounded by a single layer of cells with microvilli extending from their inner surface. When the gland is stimulated the acinar cells are columnar and the colloid is reduced but when a follicle is inactive the cells are flat and colloid accumulates. The thyroid also contains the parafollicular or 'C' cells which secrete calcitonin.

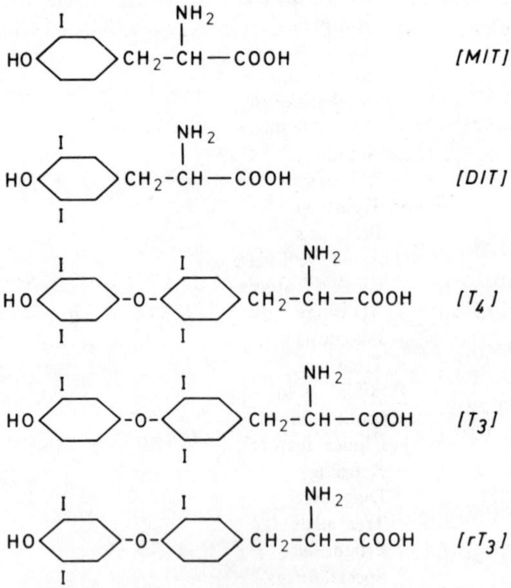

FIG. 6.1. Thyroid hormones and their precursors.

MIT = 3,–Monoiodotyrosine.
DIT = 3,5–Diiodotyrosine.
T_4 = 3,5,3′,5′–L–Tetraiodothyronine.
T_3 = 3,5,3′–L–Triiodothyronine.
rT_3 = reverse T_3 = 3,3′,5′–L–Triiodothyronine.

PHYSIOLOGY

Metabolism of iodine

The normal intake of iodine is about 1.2 μmol (150 μg) per day and the unavoidable loss is 10–20% of that. The plasma level of inorganic iodine is about 25 nmol/l (0.3 μg/100 ml). The thyroid iodide transport system is highly efficient and normally removes about 50% of the iodide from the blood passing through the gland producing a concentration gradient ranging from 25 to several hundred fold. The exact process is not understood but the transport system into the acinar cells is shared by other monovalent anions. After entry into the cell, the iodide is oxidised almost immediately and then attached to tyrosine which is already in a thyroprotein molecule. Mono- (MIT) and di-iodotyrosine (DIT) are formed (Fig. 6.1). The thyroid hormones are produced probably by coupling of MIT and DIT to form Thyroxine (T_4) and Triiodothyronine (T_3). Other iodinated compounds may be formed but they are biologically inactive. The various iodine compounds are stored in the colloid in proteins of high molecular weight, before being released into the circulation by a process of digestion and reabsorption.

'Reverse' T_3 (Fig. 6.1) is biologically inert. It can be formed readily by the fetal thyroid and peripheral conversion from T_4.

Metabolism of thyroid hormones

About 90% of the organic iodide released from the thyroid into the blood is in the form of T_4 and the rest is T_3. Most tissues have the capacity to deiodinate T_4 to T_3 or reverse T_3 (rT_3). This dual pathway constitutes a control system by diverting T_4 into a highly potent or alternatively an inactive metabolite. The ratio of T_3 to T_4 in the plasma is relatively constant despite varying thyroid function, with certain exceptions (see below). Shortly after release the thyroid hormones are bound almost entirely to plasma proteins, namely:

Thyroxine binding globulin (TBG).
Thyroxine binding pre-albumin (TBPA).
Albumin.

Various aspects of the metabolism of the two hormones are set out in Table 6.1. T_3 is more potent than T_4 on a weight basis and acts more quickly when administered, but qualitatively the two hormones have the same effects. It is not certain what proportion of thyroid hormone action on the tissues is delivered by each hormone.

TABLE 6.1. Normal values of thyroid hormones

	'T$_4$'	'T$_3$'
Plasma concentration		
Total (nmol/l)	50–150	1.5–3.0
% unbound	0.04	0.3
Free (pmol/l)	40	7
Disposal rate (adult)		
(nmol/day)	110	35
Half life in plasma	6 days	1 day
Protein binding in plasma TBG	75%	75%
TBPA	15%	?
Albumin	10%	?

Probably the hormones are destroyed in many tissues but the fate of the organic core of the molecules is uncertain. Some T$_4$ is excreted in the bile. Presumably it is the unbound hormone fraction in the plasma which equilibrates with the tissues. The free hormones enter cells and bind to receptors on the nucleus causing an increase in synthesis of certain proteins. The main overall effect is to stimulate calorigenesis but many other independent effects occur, e.g. on growth and brain function.

Control of thyroid function

Thyroid function does not depend on nutritional factors except for iodine, deficiency of which tends to cause a goitre. Thyroid function is stimulated by thyrotrophin (TSH) from the anterior pituitary. TSH secretion is in turn suppressed by the thyroid hormones in the plasma forming a self-regulating system. It is not known whether T$_3$ or T$_4$ is more important physiologically in this respect but certainly the administration of either suppresses TSH secretion.

THYROID TESTS

There is no single test which can be used to the exclusion of all others and it is important to use the tests appropriate to various circumstances. There are five types of tests:

Circulating hormones
Thyroid gland activity
Tissue function
Autoantibodies
Dynamic tests

Circulating hormones

Thyroxine
The standard test is a measurement of thyroxine in plasma, the normal level being about 50–150 nmol/l (4–12 μg/100 ml). The assay may be done using commercially prepared kits or by materials assembled locally. The principle of the test uses competitive protein binding by the equilibration of radioactive iodide-labelled hormone between a synthetic material (e.g. Sephadex) and natural plasma binding proteins in the presence of hormone extracted from the test plasma. A true radioimmunoassay is available also. The T_4 assay is of reasonable accuracy but the hormone level may be depressed by the administration of drugs including phenothiazines, phenytoin, salicylates, tolbutamide and fenclofenac. The T_4 level is influenced by the level of binding protein present and this may be increased particularly by pregnancy and the administration of oestrogens (e.g. oral contraceptives), clofibrate and perphenazone, giving misleadingly high results. Binding proteins may be depressed by androgens, anabolic steroids and corticosteroids.

It is possible to compensate for changes in binding proteins by taking a ratio of the T_4 level and an estimate of the binding capacity of the patient's plasma. The latter may be measured simply by an 'uptake test' (or 'binding test', T_3B) in which radioisotope labelled T_3 is equilibrated between the patient's plasma and another hormone binding substance. The test is sometimes called a 'T_3 test' which is unfortunate as it does not measure T_3. An 'uptake test' is influenced also by the level of circulating T_4 and has been used as a screening test, but it is much more useful as a correction factor for the T_4. The result is called a 'Free Thyroxine Index' (FTI). This is particularly useful in assessing borderline results.

Free thyroxine
The plasma thyroxine which is unbound can now be measured as a routine. It may replace total thyroxine as the standard test.

Tri-iodothyronine
Plasma T_3 can be measured by radioimmunoassay. It is particularly useful if the gland is damaged (see below).

T_3/T_4 ratio
In normal persons and in the large majority of patients with thyroid disease the ratio of T_3 to T_4 in the plasma is approximately constant so

that a measure of either may be used in assessment. Sometimes the proportion of T_3 is increased and patients may be hyperthyroid with normal levels of T_4 ('T_3 toxicosis'—see below) so that only a measurement of T_3 will confirm the diagnosis. It seems to be the case that when the function of the thyroid is impaired there is a tendency for more T_3 to be released than T_4. This can be regarded as a compensatory mechanism to make more efficient use of iodine and hormone synthesis. This situation may arise in glands after partial resection, after radioiodine treatment, in thyroiditis or iodine deficiency. In these circumstances the T_4 may be lower than the clinical state would suggest and thyroid hormone action in the tissues is maintained by a relatively higher level of T_3.

Thyroid binding proteins
These can be measured directly and may replace the present 'T_3B' tests.

Thyrotrophin (TSH)
The measurement of plasma TSH by radioimmunoassay is useful in confirming primary thyroid failure (a high level), in monitoring replacement therapy with T_4 (see below) and in conjunction with TRH (see below).

Thyroid gland function

The only means of studying thyroid gland function directly is by measuring the way it handles radioisotopes. The conventional test measures the uptake of ^{131}I into the gland 24 h after an oral dose and also examines the turnover ^{131}I through the gland during the next few days. Shorter half-life isotopes of radioiodine can be used to assess uptake over periods of 2–8 h.

Thyroid scanning
Technecium (99 Tc^m) or radioiodine given in somewhat larger doses may be used to record a thyroid 'scan'. This can be helpful in revealing the true outline of the gland, the level of function of adenomas and the presence of ectopic thyroid tissue or metastases.

Tissue function

In theory the ideal way to assess thyroid function would be to determine whether thyroid hormone-dependent tissue function was normal. The classical test of Basal Metabolic Rate was an attempt at this but has been abandoned in practice because of its expense and unreliability. An alternative is reflex timing. This makes use of the physical sign that the speed of the tendon reflexes, particularly in the relaxation phase, is related to the level of thyroid hormones, i.e. fast reflexes in *hyper*-thyroidism and slow reflexes in *hypo*thyroidism. The ankle jerk may be recorded (Fig. 6.2) but the precision of the method is not high.

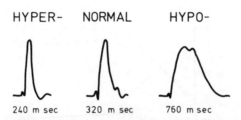

HYPER-   NORMAL   HYPO-

240 m sec   320 m sec   760 m sec

FIG. 6.2. Typical recordings by photomotograph of movement of the foot when the Achilles tendon reflex is elicited. The timing is in milliseconds from the moment of impact to half relaxation.

Thyroid autoantibodies

Both humoral and cell mediated autoimmune reactions are implicated in thyroid disease and a number of circulating thyroid autoantibodies can be detected.

The tests most commonly used are for thyroglobulin and microsomal antibodies. There is no absolute level of significance and the results vary to some extent between laboratories. In general, the tests are negative in normal persons, but positive results at low titres become increasingly common after middle age. A high titre is usual in Hashimoto's disease.

Thyroid stimulating immunoglobulins

React with and stimulate the surface receptors for TSH. The term includes substances described before as long-acting thyroid stimulator (LATS) and human specific thyroid stimulator (or LATS protector). Analysis for them is not generally available and their value in clinical practice is uncertain. Their role in the pathogenesis of hyperthyroidism is discussed below.

Dynamic tests

Older tests such as TSH stimulation, T_3 suppression and iodine loading are now rarely used but the 'TRH' test is useful.

TRH test

A slow intravenous injection of synthetic Thyrotrophin Releasing Hormone (TRH) 200 μg (for an adult) is given. The plasma TSH level is estimated just before the injection and afterwards at 20 and 60 min. In hyperthyroidism and in most euthyroid patients with thyroid eye disease, TSH response is lost and the TSH level does not rise. In hypothyroidism there is an exaggerated response (Fig. 6.3).

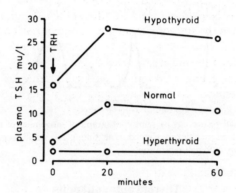

FIG. 6.3. Typical response of plasma TSH after i.v. TRH 200 mg.

THYROID DISEASES

Except for diabetes and infertility, thyroid disease is by far the commonest type of endocrine disease which is encountered. There seems to be a genetic element and about 50% of patients will have a positive family history for thyroid disease of some kind. The conditions are much commoner in women than men with a ratio of about 4:1 for hyperthyroidism and 10:1 for hypothyroidism. All ages are affected, with hyperthyroidism more common in early adult life and hypothyroidism more common in the elderly.

Goitre

A goitre (enlargement of the thyroid gland) does not necessarily indicate abnormal thyroid function, nor does its absence exclude it.

Examination of the thyroid gland

The apparent size of the gland at first sight depends on the length and shape of the patient's neck and the patient's fatness. Careful inspection of the front of the neck while the patient swallows gives a more accurate impression. Palpation of the gland should be done from in front and from behind the patient—usually the latter is more informative. The hands are placed round the neck from behind with the thumbs on the back of the neck and the finger-tips meeting in front over the trachea. The isthmus is defined first and then the lateral lobes. The patient is asked to swallow, if necessary with a sip of water, while the gland is palpated. The gland should move with the larynx during swallowing and this helps the fingers to differentiate the gland from other structures. When the sternomastoid muscles are large it may be difficult to feel the lateral lobes— it is helpful to press the thumb and finger-tips in on either side of the muscle.

The size, shape and position of the gland should be noted. It is necessary to define its consistency, regularity, mobility and attachment to related structures. The lower border should be identified to exclude a retrosternal extension. A systolic or continuous murmur may be heard over the goitre indicating increased blood flow and the likelihood of hyperthyroidism. Transmitted bruits from carotid atheroma or the aortic valve can usually be distinguished by their location. Plain radiography will reveal a retrosternal extension or tracheal compression; ultrasound will show whether the goitre is solid or cystic; laryngoscopy may show a vocal cord palsy.

Types of goitre

Physiological
The gland tends to enlarge during puberty and pregnancy. Sometimes the enlargement is sufficient to cause concern to the patient although such goitres are of moderate size only; smooth, soft and regular. No treatment is required provided that the patient is euthyroid. The gland tends to return to its normal size.

'Simple' goitre
Also sometimes called sporadic, diffuse or colloid goitre. Slight to moderate symmetrical enlargement of the thyroid, particularly in women, is quite common. The patients are euthyroid and not iodine deficient. The goitres persist over many years and may become multinodular. The prognosis is uncertain; neoplasia is unlikely but hyperthyroidism may develop. The aetiology of simple goitre is unknown. Treatment with thyroxine is recommended sometimes but seems ineffective. Surgery may be required if the goitre gets very large.

Iodine deficiency
In some areas remote from the sea the iodine content of the soil is so low that iodine deficiency may occur in isolated communities eating only locally produced food. When the daily intake falls below about 400 nmol (50 μg) per day a considerable proportion of the population develop a compensatory goitre which may later become multinodular. In some areas there may be a genetic effect also. The individuals are euthyroid but their babies may be cretinous. Iodine dietary supplements are effective but may increase the incidence of hyperthyroidism. There is no recent epidemiological data but probably iodine deficiency goitre does not now occur in the UK and our table salt is not iodised.

Thyrotoxic goitre
See below under hyperthyroidism.

Enzyme defects
There are a number of rare genetically determined biochemical defects in the thyroid all of which cause defective thyroid hormone synthesis (dyshormonogenesis). There is a goitre and hypothyroidism which may be present from birth or develop during childhood. The defects include:

Iodide trapping defect (very rare)
Iodide binding defects
Iodide binding defect with congenital nerve deafness (Pendred's syndrome)
Abnormal circulating iodine containing proteins.

Neoplasm

Benign
The commonest tumour of the thyroid is the benign adenoma, which may be cystic. The tumours may be single or multiple and may arise in a previously normal gland or in one which is hypertrophied. The aetiology is unknown. The histology may be classified into different types but clinically, only two types are recognised, the 'hot', i.e. active, and 'cold'. The differentiation can be made clinically only by a radioisotope scan to show whether the adenoma is concentrating isotope or not. If it is, the activity tends to escape from physiological control and hyperthyroidism ensues. The rising level of thyroid hormone suppresses the secretion of TSH so that the rest of the gland becomes inactive. With a 'cold' adenoma the rest of the gland maintains normal func-

tion. Malignant change in 'hot' adenomas is very rare but there is debate about the incidence of malignancy in 'cold' adenomas and based on the histological appearance widely differing figures are given. The clinical impression is that malignant change is rare. Cystic adenomas are usually, but unfortunately not always, benign.

Treatment. A small indolent asymptomatic adenoma may be treated conservatively, particularly in the elderly. If the adenoma is enlarging or if any characteristics suggestive of malignancy arise, it should be removed. In general, because of the remote risk of malignancy, cold adenomas should be removed. It is said that if adenomas are multiple, malignancy is unlikely but histology indicates that they are in fact usually multiple even if this is not apparent clinically. Large multiple adenomas may require removal for cosmetic reasons or because of pressure symptoms. The solitary 'hot' nodule causing hyperthyroidism can be removed but it can be treated medically in the usual way if surgery is contra-indicated.

Malignant

These are nearly always carcinomas. Secondary tumour is not rare but usually it is discovered by routine examination at autopsy. Primary carcinoma of the thyroid is uncommon and accounts for less than 0.5% of all deaths due to carcinoma.

Clinical features. Initial diagnosis depends on physical examination. Features of a goitre which raise the suspicion of malignancy are:

Vocal cord paralysis
Attachment to surrounding tissues
Rapid increase in size
Hardness
Pressure symptoms
Immobility

All these features may mislead but the first two are the most reliable. Thyroid carcinomas are classified as:

Papillary. This is the commonest form. It occurs in children and the middle-aged. It spreads to regional lymph nodes but is often resectable and has a good prognosis.

Follicular. This is the next commonest and tends to arise later in life. Blood-borne metastases may occur but following surgery and suppressive T_4 the prognosis is fair.

Anaplastic. This is less common, and tends to arise in the elderly. It is a highly malignant tumour; usually surgery is impossible and the prognosis is bad.

Medullary. This is the rarest thyroid carcinoma and arises in young adults. The tumour secretes calcitonin and other hormones. High plasma levels of calcitonin are a specific tumour marker but do not produce changes in plasma calcium. The tumour may be familial in association with other endocrine tumours. The prognosis is fair.

Treatment. This is by resection if possible followed by radiotherapy. The relatively well-differentiated thyroid carcinomas may have the capacity to take up iodine and this is useful in therapy with large doses of radioiodine. Subsequently, thyroxine is given in a dose sufficient to depress the plasma TSH to unrecordable levels. This treatment is continued indefinitely to discourage recurrence.

Inflammation

Autoimmune thyroiditis (Hashimoto's disease, lymphadenoid goitre).

Clinical features. This condition presents usually with a slowly enlarging, symmetrical, regular, firm, moderate sized goitre in a middle-aged woman. The gland may be painful and tender. The patient may be euthyroid or hypothyroid or, more rarely, hyperthyroid. The nature of the goitre may raise the suspicion of malignancy. Thyroid antibodies are almost always present in high titre.

Pathology. The histology is variable but includes diffuse lymphocytic infiltration, obliteration of thyroid follicles and fibrosis. Some epithelial cells are larger with oxyphilic changes in the cytoplasm (Askanazy cells). Attempts to differentiate various types have been made.

Diagnosis. Can only be made conclusively by histology but thyroid biopsy is not practised often as it is unreliable, and operation should be avoided. A presumptive diagnosis can be made on the clinical features with high antibodies. Isotope uptake may be raised, normal or low. In many patients thiocyanate will discharge some radioiodine from the gland after it has been taken up.

Treatment. If the gland is large it may be necessary to remove it but this should be avoided as the gland tends to shrink with time. Thyroxine treatment may accelerate this and will be needed anyway in hypothyroid patients. Hypothyroidism ensues eventually in many patients but this may be delayed for years. Hyperthyroidism is best managed with antithyroid drugs.

Subacute granulomatous thyroiditis (de Quervain's disease)
This is an uncommon disease due perhaps to a virus infection. The gland is painful, tender and swollen; there are minor systemic symptoms but no change in thyroid function. Thyroid antibodies are absent. The disease is self-limiting but corticosteroid treatment may ease pain.

Fibrous thyroiditis (Riedel's disease)
This very rare disease of unknown aetiology produces an intense fibrosis of the gland which may reproduce pressure symptoms. The hardness of the gland suggests carcinoma but the process is benign.

Pyogenic thyroiditis
This may occur from infection with any pyogenic organism but it is a rare complication even in severe septicaemia.

HYPERTHYROIDISM

This is the condition in which the action of the thyroid hormones on the tissues is excessive. Mild degrees of it are only a quantitative deviation from normal and the dividing line between euthyroid and hyperthyroid is arbitrary. In more severe forms definitely pathological features appear. There is no good reason to use the word 'thyrotoxicosis' to mean anything other than 'hyperthyroidism'.

Clinical features

In some patients with hyperthyroidism the features are so obvious that the diagnosis can be made at a glance but there are many variants and the disease may be cryptic. The effect on various systems of the same degree of thyroid overactivity varies surprisingly from patient to patient.

Symptoms
The onset may be over a few weeks or be quite insidious. The commonest symptoms are nervousness, sweating, palpitations, fatigue and weight loss, despite a good appetite. Other symptoms include intoler-

ance of heat, tremor, insomnia, frequent stools or diarrhoea, and dyspnoea. The patient may have noticed eye changes and neck swelling. In elderly patients lassitude and cardiovascular symptoms are particularly common.

Physical examination
The fully developed clinical picture is striking. The patient is thin, abnormally alert, and restless; movements are quick and impulsive. The eyes are wide open (the so-called 'thyrotoxic glitter') and the neck is full. The skin is of fine texture, flushed, warm and sweating, the pulse is fast and the pulse pressure increased. However, the features are diverse; it is impossible to compose a clinical picture which is always reliable and there are many exceptions. For example, the appetite may increase so much that the body weight is maintained or even increased. There may be no eye changes particularly in the elderly. The change in mental state may be so great as to produce a psychosis and mental hospital admission. The diarrhoea may be so severe as to be the presenting feature and suggest a colitis. The spleen may be just palpable.

The neck. Some enlargement of the thyroid is almost always present— some would say always—and the difference depends perhaps on the definition of the upper limit of normal. Certainly, in the elderly the enlargement may be very slight. Typically, the enlargement is generalised and symmetrical but often the gland is nodular or contains an adenoma. A bruit over the gland is confirmatory evidence of overactivity.

Nervous system. Some patients comment on a desire for extra activity but others have lassitude and are easily fatigued. Some patients complain of specific muscle weakness and there may be a proximal myopathy with wasting, particularly of the shoulder girdle. There is usually a fine tremor of the outstretched hands and occasionally the tremor is gross and disabling. Athetosis may occur. The tendon reflexes are brisk, often on slight impact, and the speed of the muscle movement tends to be increased.

Cardiovascular system. The sitting pulse may be 120/min or more and often the sleeping pulse is raised. The apex beat is forceful to maintain the hyperdynamic circulation and a systolic murmur from increased flow may be heard but unless heart failure occurs the heart is of normal size clinically and normal also by radiography and electrocardiography.

Sometimes, particularly in the elderly, more serious changes ensue. The commonest is auricular fibrillation, which is the same in all respects as that occurring from other causes, except that it may revert to sinus rhythm when the thyroid is controlled. Congestive cardiac failure may occur and indeed this may be the only major feature of hyperthyroidism, posing a considerable diagnostic problem. It is likely that much of the increased incidence of cardiovascular changes in hyperthyroidism in the elderly is due to coexistent ischaemic heart disease.

'T_3' Thyrotoxicosis

This term is applied to the small proportion of patients (? 2%) with hyperthyroidism who have normal levels of plasma T_4 but raised T_3. It is important to emphasise that the general clinical features are exactly the same whether the excess hormone is T_3 or T_4 and the significance of the condition lies only in the interpretation of the tests.

Thyroid storm (Thyrotoxic crisis)

This uncommon condition is a sudden gross exacerbation of severe hyperthyroidism. The patient becomes restless and later semicomatose. The pulse rate rises to 150–200/min and the body temperature to 39° or more. Heart failure and death may ensue; urgent treatment is imperative. Thyroid storm occurs in the neglected patient with florid disease or after sub-total thyroidectomy in a patient who has not been made euthyroid before surgery and is due presumably to a sudden further leakage of thyroid hormone into the circulation. A thyroid storm represents a failure in management.

Pathology and aetiology

The histology of the thyroid gland in hyperthyroidism is variable. The acini contain a reduced amount of colloid and the epithelial cells are tall and crowded. There is increased vascularity and lymphocytic infiltration with increased fibrous tissue may be seen. If there is a hyperactive adenoma that may have any of the various histological patterns and the rest of the gland will be inactive.

Many uncertainties still surround the aetiology of hyperthyroidism but its occurrence implies that the hormone secretion is no longer TSH dependent. If there is inflammation in the gland there is presumably tissue destruction and release of hormone. In an adenoma the tissue is biochemically incomplete in that hormone synthesis occurs but the normal control is reduced. In the commonest form of hyperthyroidism, i.e. Graves' disease with a diffusely hyperplastic gland, it seems likely that there is some process stimulating the tissue. Probably all patients with Graves' disease have a 'thyroid stimulating immunoglobulin' (TSI) in the plasma (see above). Factors influencing the production of TSI are unknown but it seems that in untreated Graves' disease the system is to some extent self-perpetuating because after treatment with antithyroid drugs only half the patients with Graves' disease still have TSI and after sub-total thyroidectomy the proportion is about 15%. The only factor known to precipitate hyperthyroidism is iodine supplementation in iodine deficient areas. There is an impression that hyperthyroidism may follow emotional stress but this is unproven.

In many patients there is a family history of thyroid disease or autoimmune disorder such as pernicious anaemia. The genetic component may be mediated by an inherited capacity to produce TSI.

Diagnosis

It should be possible to reach a correct clinical diagnosis in hyperthyroidism in at least 80% of patients but it is not easy to say how it should be done. Attempts have been made to produce diagnostic indices by adding together numerical scores for the various features of the condition but they have not been particularly successful and none have been adopted generally. Best guidance is obtained from the history, the patients general appearance and behaviour, the neck, eyes, and cardiovascular system. It is prudent to include at least one biochemical test and the best currently available is the plasma T_4 or T_3, preferably coupled with some correction for protein binding. In case of difficulty a TRH test may help. In the borderline case a period of observation and repeat testing is valuable—little is lost by not reaching an immediate diagnosis.

Problems
The differentiation from an anxiety state may be difficult because both conditions share many features. Reliance may have to be placed on biochemical tests. Hyperthyroidism in the elderly may be cryptic and present in the form of auricular fibrillation and/or congestive cardiac failure with few other signs, and, rarely, with withdrawal and apathy. Occasionally, psychotic patients, particularly those with agitation and tremor, may be hyperthyroid. In pregnancy and in women on oestrogens the thyroid hormone levels are raised and the results must be corrected for the changes in binding proteins.

T_4 measurements may be changed by drug administration. The interpretation of thyroid function tests must include a consideration of the individual patient with particular reference to medication and previous thyroid disease and treatment. Possible changes in T_3/T_4 ratio as described above in the section on thyroid tests should be borne in mind if the clinical appearances are discordant with the T_4 results.

Treatment

The treatment of hyperthyroidism is only moderately satisfactory. There are four main methods used often in combination.

Symptomatic
β-adrenergic blocking drugs achieve rapid control of some of the troublesome symptoms of severe hyperthyroidism such as palpitations, sweating and tremor. These drugs have little effect on thyroid function and should not be used in the long term nor if the symptoms above are absent. Mild sedatives may be helpful also.

Iodine
This has no effect on a normal person but in hyperthyroidism its administration suppresses thyroid hormone release. The effect is incomplete and transient, so that iodine has no place in long-term management. It is useful in preparation for surgery (see below). Treatment is given by mouth with aqueous iodine solution (Lugol's) 0.5 ml (65 mg of iodine) each day.

Theocarbamides
This is the main group of drugs in use; the earlier thiouracils have been largely replaced by *carbimazole*. Thiocarbamides act by suppressing several stages of the synthesis of thyroid hormones. The dose has to be adjusted to the individual—carbimazole, 10 mg three times a day by mouth is an appropriate starting dose for an adult but this may have to be doubled. The overall effect is slow and the patients may not become euthyroid until they have been treated for 3–5 weeks, but thereafter it is sometimes possible to reduce the dose progressively to about 10 mg a day. β-adrenergic blocking drugs (e.g. propranolol 20 to 40 mg three times a day) are a useful adjunct at first in the severe case. The side effects of thiocarbamides are infrequent but may be severe. Gastric upset may be dealt with by a change to propyl thiouracil. Sensitivity rashes may occur but more serious is the agranulocytosis which may affect patients during the first few weeks of treatment. This complication is an unpredictable idiosyncrasy and occurs without warning, probably in less than 1% of patients. Routine white cell counts are not helpful and should not be done. It is more important to warn the patient to report at once any sore throat, fever or malaise.

Potassium perchlorate has an antithyroid action by blocking the iodide trap. It is a useful alternative if there is an adverse reaction to the thiocarbamides although it has similar risks.

Management of treatment
It can be difficult to adjust the dose of carbimazole correctly. Some physicians use large doses continuously and add thyroxine to keep the patient euthyroid. The effect of treatment is best judged by the relief of the patient's symptoms and their return to their own normal weight; biochemical tests are of limited use only. Persistent elevation of T_4 indicates inadequate suppression but satisfactory treatment may be accompanied by low levels of T_4. If the response is favourable, the gland may diminish in size with time but this is not always the case. Treatment should be continued for 18–24 months and then discontinued. About 50% of the patients will stay in remission but the others relapse and a further decision must be taken about therapy—usually radioiodine or surgery is recommended. Despite many attempts no satisfactory test is available to predict at the outset which patients will relapse when treatment is stopped.

Radioiodine
Because thyroid tissue traps and retains iodine, radiation damage of the gland can be produced by a dose of radioiodine which gives only trivial radiation to other tissues. The dose is usually in the range of 2 to 6 mCi of ^{131}I given as carrier free iodide in water as a drink.

The dose may be adjusted to allow for the size of the gland and its rate of iodine uptake but such adjustments do not help much and we now use a standard dose of 5 mCi for al patients. There is no systemic disturbance but there may be transient swelling and tenderness of the gland. Thyroid function declines slowly over several months. In an attempt to reduce the incidence of late hypothyroidism (see below) relatively small doses are usual nowadays but often they are inadequate and repeated doses are needed. Two days after the dose of radioiodine, thiocarbamides should be started and maintained as necessary. Previous iodine treatment renders radioiodine ineffective by preventing uptake. Thiocarbamides have to be withdrawn for at least 48 h before radioiodine can be used.

Radioiodine treatment is believed to carry no appreciable risk of carcinogenesis in the thyroid or elsewhere. Because of possible genetic hazards it should not be given to women or men under the age of 45 years. The main problem with radioiodine treatment is the later occurrence of hypothyroidism. The incidence of this may be as high as 40% after ten years and continues to rise slowly thereafter. For this reason long-term follow up is essential after radioactive iodine treatment. This problem has reduced the value of radioiodine because the use of lower doses has extended the time necessary to control the disease. One suggestion is to use ablating doses of radioiodine and accept hypothyroidism as inevitable from the outset.

Surgery
The operation is that of sub-total thyroidectomy. Usually, about $\frac{7}{8}$ of the gland is removed with special attention to preservation of the parathyroid glands and the recurrent laryngeal nerves. The preparation of the patients is important and they must be rendered euthyroid with thiocarbamide or iodine before operation. Some surgeons prefer thiocarbamide followed by iodine alone for the last two weeks before surgery to reduce the vascularity of the gland. Thyroid surgery is relatively specialised and is best left in the hands of those with special interest and experience. The mortality rate is very low but tetany may occur from parathyroid damage. Later difficulties are recurrence of hyperthyroidism (about 5%) and hypothyroidism (perhaps 10%). Repeat operations are to be avoided. The success of the operation is unexplained. It seems that the removal of the larger part of the toxic gland interrupts the underlying pathological process and permits the remaining tissue to return to normal physiological control.

Selection of treatment for hyperthyroidism

Thiocarbamide, radioiodine or surgery?
Sometimes there are factors which make selection obvious but often there is a choice. Some of the pros and cons are set out in Table 6.2.

The following rules of selection seem satisfactory although they show a physician's bias to medical treatment.
1. If there is a diffuse goitre, thiocarbamide is given for 18–24 months perhaps with propranolol at first.
2. In the elderly patients with diffuse goitre, radioiodine is given first and then thiocarbamide.
3. If there are one or more adenomas, a large goitre, tracheal compression, rapid enlargement or retrosternal extension and the patient's general condition is good, surgery is advised.
4. If the control with thiocarbamide is poor, if sensitivity occurs or if there is relapse after stopping thiocarbamide, surgery is advised in the younger patient and radioiodine in the older.
5. If there is relapse after surgery, or if the patient refuses other forms of treatment, thiocarbamide is used, if necessary indefinitely.

TABLE 6.2. Factors in the selection of treatment for hyperthyroidism

	Thiocarbamide	Radioiodine	Surgery
For	Out-patient 50% remission	Out-patient No mortality Painless Useful in poor risk patients	High cure rate Removes goitre
	Useful in poor risk patients		Relieves pressure Quick
Against	50% relapse	May need repeated doses	Hospitalisation

	Continued treatment
	  and supervision
	  needed
		Hypothyroidism	Scar
			Complications

	Adverse reactions	Genetic risk	Mortality (slight)

Special circumstances

Pregnancy. The problem is not common as hyperthyroidism reduces fertility but treatment may be followed by conception—patients should be warned of this and suitable contraceptive advice given if treatment is continuing. There is no general agreement as to the best treatment of hyperthyroidism in pregnancy. If the condition is mild, treatment may be withheld, at least in the first few weeks but this may increase the risk of miscarriage. Thiocarbamides are believed to be non-teratogenic and may be used. As the end of the pregnancy approaches the dose should be reduced to a minimum as the drug crosses the placenta and can produce a goitre in the fetus. Radioiodine is contra-indicated.

Thyroid storm. This life threatening condition demands immediate vigorous treatment. β-adrenergic blocking drugs are the most important therapy and should be given intravenously in full doses. A large dose of carbimazole (e.g. 100 mg) by mouth or stomach tube should be given at once. Intravenous hydrocortisone and iodine have been recommended. Hyperpyrexia is controlled by exposure; supportive therapy with oxygen, intravenous fluids and drugs for heart failure may be needed.

Prognosis

The natural history of hyperthyroidism depends on the aetiology. If there is a thyroiditis remission is certain but is likely to be followed by hypothyroidism. A toxic adenoma is unlikely to revert and requires surgery. Graves' disease runs an intermittent course. Sometimes it will remit spontaneously after a short illness. Under treatment with thio-carbamide about 50% of patients remit within two years but further episodes of hyperthyroidism may occur. Death from hyperthyroidism is rare and the operative mortality is less than 1%. The prognosis after surgery and radioiodine is described above.

THYROID EYE DISEASE

Clinical features

The majority of patients with hyperthyroidism have some changes in the eyes, but these changes are not exclusive to thyroid overactivity—they may occur also in euthyroid persons and rarely even in hypo-thyroidism. The changes are usually bilateral but often asymmetrical and in a few patients the changes are confined to one eye. Changes within the eye include papilloedema and optic atrophy but such risk to sight is rare.

The nomenclature is unsatisfactory—the terms 'exophthalmos' or 'endocrine exophthalmos' are used but there is no relationship to any endocrine gland except the thyroid and exophthalmos is only part of the condition. Four main components can be distinguished; they may occur almost independently of each other. Even in combination, the degree of each may differ although all are likely to be present in the severe case. The severity varies from the trivial to the catastrophic. The four components are:

Lid retraction
This affects particularly the upper lid and may be more obvious when the patient's eyes move from horizontal to downwards gaze (lid lag). Lid retraction can be detected by looking at the relationship between the iris and the edges of the eye lids. If all the iris margin can be seen lid retraction is present.

Soft tissue inflammation
This is a sterile inflammation of the conjunctivae and the soft tissues of the eyelids. The conjunctivae become injected and the patient com-plains of irritation and a gritty sensation in the eyes. Lacrimation is increased but there is no pus and the eyelids are not stuck together on waking. The eyelids may be swollen. Sometimes the conjunctival vessels become considerably enlarged.

Exophthalmos
This is due to an increase in the bulk of the muscles and other tissue in the retro-orbital space. The eye ball is pushed forwards, usually by 2–3 mm, but sometimes more. The degree of exophthalmos may be judged by inspecting the eye ball from the side and the degree of protrusion can be measured by an exophthalmometer.

Weakness of the extraocular muscles
In the mild case this causes a diplopia, perhaps on looking in a particular direction or maybe when the patient is tired. Any or all of the muscles may be involved and in the more severe examples there is an obvious strabismus, and, very rarely, complete ophthalmoplegia.

Natural history
This condition usually appears as hyperthyroidism develops. Control of the hyperthyroidism is likely to be followed by a rather slow improvement in the eye changes but this is by no means always so and the eyes may get progressively worse over weeks or months. After a few months the condition tends to stabilise and thereafter there is slow improvement. Eventually complete remission can be virtually guaranteed but this may take 3–5 years and some residual exophthalmos may remain.

Aetiology and pathology

The cause of thyroid eye disease is unknown. An 'exophthalmos producing substance' has been described but its significance is uncertain. Thyroid stimulating immunoglobulins may be involved. The increase in bulk of the retro-ocular tissue is due to oedema caused by an increase of hydrophilic material in the connective tissue. The changes in the extraocular muscles appears to be a primary myopathy with inflammatory changes, increase in connective tissue and fatty infiltration.

Diagnosis

This is always made on clinical grounds as there is no specific test. When hyperthyroidism is present the diagnosis will be obvious. If the patient is euthyroid it may be possible to implicate thyroid disease by the loss of TSH response after TRH. The most difficult situation is with unilateral exophthalmos when it is essential to exclude other orbital conditions such as tumour. Extensive investigations with radiography and scanning techniques may be required because the diagnosis is reached by exclusion.

Treatment

The management of thyroid eye disease is difficult and unsatisfactory. The patient may well find that the eye symptoms are the worst part of the thyroid illness. It is important to explain the situation to the patient at the outset and stress that control of the gland will not necessarily help the eyes, that there is no cure for the eye disease, that eventual remission, perhaps after years, is almost certain and that there is virtually no danger to sight.

Diplopia may be helped by an eye patch and methyl cellulose eye drops will ease the discomfort. β-adrenergic blocking drugs seem to have no effect and our experience of guanethidine eye drops has not been encouraging. The eyes should be observed carefully and frequently if exophthalmos is progressive because it may reach a point where the eyelids no longer meet on blinking and this exposes the cornea to the danger of drying out and ulceration; tarsorraphy is then indicated. This minor operation involves stitching together the outer ends of the eyelids to effectively shorten the length of the palpebral fissure and draw the eyelids together. The eyelids can be separated again later when the condition subsides. For severe cases operation to decompress the orbit by removing part of its wall and some of the retro-ocular tissue may be necessary. Medically, the only drugs reported to be of use are corticosteroids in large doses and these should be reserved for the severe case. It is debatable what effect the treatment of the hyperthyroidism has on the eye disease and no particular therapy seems advantageous in this respect. It is considered that too rapid suppression of thyroid function and hypothyroidism are to be avoided.

PRETIBIAL MYXOEDEMA

This uncommon condition occurs in patients with Graves' disease, usually with eye changes. The lesion is a red or violaceous induration of the skin, with infiltration by mucopolysaccharide over the pretibial area. It runs an indolent course but may respond to treatment with local steroids.

HYPOTHYROIDISM

This is the condition in which the action of thyroid hormones on the tissues is deficient. The same considerations of the borderline between normal and abnormal apply as in hyperthyroidism. 'Myxoedema' should refer to the deposition of myxoedematous material in the tissues and is sometimes used to mean gross clinical hypothyroidism but usually the term is taken as equivalent to hypothyroidism.

Clinical features

The onset is insidious in most patients and may escape notice by those who see the patient frequently. There is likely to be a general slowing down and increasing difficulty in coping with job or home, but the presenting symptoms are variable. Common complaints are of weakness, sleepiness, lethargy, poor memory and concentration, weight gain and constipation. In addition the patient may have noticed loss of hair, dry coarse skin, swollen eyelids, changes in facial appearance and pallor. Often the voice changes, becoming slow and hoarse. The patient may complain of feeling cold or admit an intolerance of cold weather. A carpal tunnel syndrome may be present. Swelling of the feet is common and older patients may have exertional dyspnoea. Rarely, other patterns of mental change appear and even frank psychosis ('myxoedema madness'). Examination may confirm the slow mentality and gruff voice. In the severe case the facial appearance is striking but in the younger patient with mild disease the diagnosis can be difficult. The patient is likely to be overweight but not grossly obese. The skin is pale and often yellow tinged. The hands are cool and dry and the pulse tends to be slow. Serous effusions may occur into any of the body cavities. Dependent pitting oedema is common and occasionally congestive cardiac failure may be present. The tendon reflexes show a characteristic slowing, particularly of the relaxation phase. This change is seen most obviously in the ankle reflex and constitutes a valuable guide to diagnosis. In most patients the thyroid gland cannot be felt but this is not the case in Hashimoto's disease and dyshormonogenetic hypothyroidism.

Aetiology

The causes of hypothyroidism may be classified as follows:

Idiopathic
This is by far the commonest type and the cause is uncertain but the

presence of thyroid autoantibodies in many of the patients coupled with the histology of the thyroid remnant has led to the proposal that this condition is a late outcome of a form of autoimmune thyroiditis.

Radiation
Radioiodine treatment for hyperthyroidism produces hypothyroidism eventually in a high proportion of cases.

Thyroiditis
Sub-acute thyroiditis does not usually destroy the gland but Hashimoto's disease causes thyroid failure eventually in most patients.

Surgery
Neck surgery may involve unavoidable thyroid ablation. After subtotal thyroidectomy the gland remnant fails in 5–10% of patients.

Dyshormonogenesis and agenesis
These genetically determined conditions cause thyroid hormone deficiency.

Secondary
This is caused by a deficiency of TSH and forms a major part of the syndrome of panhypopituitarism. TSH secretion may fail after pituitary surgery or irradiation. An isolated spontaneous deficiency of TSH may occur but is very rare.

Iodine deficiency
It seems to be impossible to become so iodine deficient that hypothyroidism occurs but children born to women with iodine deficiency may be affected.

Lithium
This depresses thyroid function and has been used in the treatment of hyperthyroidism. Of patients treated with lithium for psychiatric disorders a small proportion become frankly hypothyroid. The biochemical cause of the thyroid failure and its natural history are unknown; there is no goitre. Thyroxine relieves the symptoms and does not interfere with the benefits of lithium treatment.

Pathology
Histology of the gland remnant will show fibrosis and sometimes

Askanazy cells as in Hashimoto's disease. In other tissues the only consistent change is the deposition of the typical mucopolysaccharide, particularly in the skin.

Diagnosis

A clinical diagnosis, however strong, should always be confirmed by laboratory tests because it is difficult or impossible to do so once therapy is established. The plasma T_4 is the best single guide. The plasma TSH is helpful also; a raised level confirms hypothyroidism if the T_4 is borderline and also excludes a secondary thyroid failure. In the doubtful case a TRH test may help. High titres of thyroid autoantibodies will indicate the aetiology but give no guide to the level of thyroid function. Usually there is a slight anaemia and sometimes a macrocytosis. Megaloblasts are not found unless there is a coexisting pernicious anaemia, which is a known association. In severe hypothyroidism typically the electrocardiogram has low voltage complexes and isoelectric or inverted T waves, but these are unreliable features in diagnosis. Occasionally, it may be necessary to make a therapeutic trial with thyroxine.

Treatment

This should be with oral L-thyroxine sodium, which is a synthetic compound stable on storage and of reliable potency. Tablets of 25, 50 and 100 micrograms are available. A recent change in specification has increased the effective strength of the tablets by about 10%. Care is needed to avoid overdosage which may occur with some of the treatment regimes recommended previously. In the mild case, particularly if the patient is not old, treatment may be started at 50 micrograms a day. This is increased to 100 micrograms per day after two weeks and then to 150 mg per day after a further two weeks. In the elderly or severe case the author prefers to give 25 mg a day for a week to begin with. This slow progression is believed to reduce the risk of myocardial infarction. As thyroxine is so slowly acting the whole daily dose should be taken together at whichever time is convenient.

The dose of 150 mg should be continued for about a month and the patient reassessed. Most patients finally settle on a dose of 150 or 200 mg per day but occasionally as little as 100 or as much as 400 mg are needed. It can be difficult to decide on the best dose. The patient's well being and return to their normal weight is the best guide. A raised plasma TSH suggests the dose is too low but the plasma T_4 is a poor guide and is of use mainly to check whether the patient is taking the tablets. Residual symptoms may of course be due to other causes. An increase in angina may make it impossible to give full replacement doses of thyroxine but β-adrenergic blockade may help. Dosage of thyroxine should not be changed frequently because of the long delay in reaching a steady state—alterations every one or two months are appropriate. Sometimes it is helpful to ask the patient to try adjusting their own dose to find the one that suits them best. When the patient is euthyroid it is important to impress on them, and if possible their relatives, that the treatment must be continued indefinitely, must not be stopped during intercurrent illness and is compatible with any other medicines which may be prescribed. An occasional missed dose does not matter. Triiodothyronine is expensive and need not be used.

Prognosis

Prolonged hypothyroidism probably accelerates atheroma so that the treated patient may be left with a legacy of arterial damage which will shorten their life but otherwise life expectancy with treatment is normal and there need be no restriction of activity. A remission of established thyroid failure is rare.

Special forms

Neonatal hypothyroidism (Cretinism)

This is hypothyroidism occurring *in utero* or early life. Thyroid hormones cross the placenta little if at all so that the fetus is dependent on its own supply. In cretinism as it occurs in the UK it seems that complete agenesis of the thyroid is uncommon and that usually there is some thyroid tissue which either fails *in utero* or is soon no longer adequate to supply the needs of the new-born child. The thyroid tissue may be ectopic. The clinical features will depend on the timing and severity of the thyroid failure—a child born with hypothyroidism is likely to have permanent brain damage whereas if the hypothyroidism arises soon after birth early treatment may allow normal brain development.

The cretinous infant is dull and apathetic with coarse facies and a hoarse cry. There may be prolonged jaundice. The tongue is large and protruding. Usually an umbilical hernia and constipation are present; the skin has changes similar to those in the hypothyroid adult. If the thyroid failure arises a little later the presentation may be insidious with slow development and constipation. A goitre is present in the dyshormonogenetic forms. '*Juvenile myxoedema*' is thyroid failure occurring during infancy or childhood after a period of normal development. The likely presentation is with slow growth and the child's trunk may be disproportionately long compared with the limbs. Radiographs of the epiphyses show a stippled appearance—these changes may arise *in utero* in the severe cretin.

The incidence of neonatal hypothyroidism is about 1:3300 live births. Biochemical screening at birth (e.g. by assay of TSH on cord blood) is possible and it is hoped that this valuable test will soon be routine. Diagnosis can be confirmed by T_4 assay and treatment is a matter of urgency. The prognosis for mental development is variable as indicated but physical development should be normal.

Myxoedema coma

Severe hypothyroidism may present with the patient in coma, often accompanied by hypothermia. The effects of the latter on the tendon reflexes and the ECG may make the clinical diagnosis of hypothyroidism difficult or impossible. If the condition is suspected blood should be taken for analysis and treatment with thyroid hormone commenced at once, in conjunction with other appropriate measures, such as slow rewarming. Opinions differ as to whether high or low doses of thyroid hormones are indicated. In such a desperate circumstance it seems reasonable to give high doses (e.g. T_3 100 mg i.v.) with hydrocortisone.

FURTHER READING

BURROW G.N. (1978). Hyperthyroidism during pregnancy. *New England Journal of Medicine,* **298,** 150.

DE GROOT L.J. & STANBURY J.B. (1975). *The Thyroid and its Diseases* (4th Edition) John Wiley and Sons, New York.

DONIACH D. & ROITT I.M. (1975). Thyroid auto-allergic disease, in *Clinical aspects of Immunology.* (3rd Edition) by Gell, Coombs and Lachmann. Blackwell Scientific Publications, Oxford.

GREIG W.R. (1973). Radioactive iodine therapy for thyrotoxicosis. *British Journal of Surgery,* **60,** 758.

HEDINGER C. (1974). Histological typing of thyroid tumours. W.H.O. Geneva.

MILLER J.M. *et al* (1979). Diagnosis of thyroid nodules. *Journal of the American Medical Association,* **241,** 481.

WERNER S.C. & INGBAR (1978). *The Thyroid.* (4th Edition) Harper and Row, London.

Chapter 7
Calcium, Bone and Parathyroid

The clinical problems related to calcium metabolism are common and various. Although some have no evident endocrine cause they are interrelated and are discussed together.

METABOLISM OF CALCIUM AND PHOSPHORUS

About 40% of the calcium in the diet is absorbed by the small intestine via a specific transport system dependent on Vitamin D. Details of the control of calcium absorption are poorly understood. Calcium is lost from the body into the urine and by secretion into the gut. The urine calcium is determined by active tubular reabsorption, stimulated by parathyroid hormone (PTH), so that only a small fraction of the filtered calcium is excreted. Urine calcium is closely proportional to plasma calcium but small changes in the latter produce large changes in the former so presumably this system has a major role in the control of plasma calcium.

The normal level of plasma calcium is, in most laboratories, 2.3 to 2.6 mmol/l (9.2 to 10.8 mg/100 ml) assuming that blood is drawn without venous stasis and with the patient fasting. The plasma calcium exists in three forms, i.e. 65% ionised, 30% bound to protein (mostly albumin) and 5% complexed to small organic molecules, such as citrate. Because of the binding a variation in plasma proteins alters the level of calcium. To make an approximate correction, increase the calcium by 0.1 mmol/l for every 6 g/l the albumin falls below 40 g/l and vice versa when the albumin is above 40 g/l.

All the body phosphorus is in some form of chemical combination, usually as phosphate, with calcium, lipids or other organic molecules. For brevity, the word 'phosphate' is used to mean inorganic or ionised phosphate. The control of phosphate metabolism is relatively coarse compared with that of calcium. About two thirds of the dietary phosphate is absorbed, probably by diffusion. The normal plasma phosphate is about 0.8 to 1.4 mmol/l (2.5–4.3 mg/100 ml) and tends to be lower after a meal. The level of plasma phosphate does not seem to be critical for cellular function—there is considerable fluctuation in normal health, greater fluctuations in disease and a major increase in renal failure. Only long-term bone metabolism seems to be effected. All the plasma phosphate is filtered by the glomerulus and there is tubular metabolism probably by reabsorption and secretion. PTH increases phosphate clearance but the total urinary phosphate is determined by intestinal absorption.

BONE STRUCTURE

Most bone has a cortex or solid outer layer and a central or medullary zone of spongy (or cancellous) bone. The latter is an irregular honeycomb of thin branching plates called trabeculae but most of the volume is the marrow cavity. The two kinds of bone have the same innate structure and chemistry. The protein basis of bone (bone matrix or osteoid tissue) is collagen fibres arranged in regular layers parallel with the surface of the trabeculae or concentrically around the Haversian canals in the cortex. Between the collagen fibres is some interstitial material, mostly polysaccharide. The bone crystals are laid down along and in the collagen fibres. The crystals are of hydroxyapatite which is a 2.2:1 mixture by weight of calcium and phosphorus plus small amounts of sodium, carbonate and other elements such as fluorine. The formation of the bone crystals depends on processes which are poorly understood but it is thought that the product of the concentrations of calcium and phosphate in the plasma is relevant.

The necessity for other factors such as vitamin D metabolites is debatable. The crystals are formed in a regular fashion next to existing crystals forming a 'calcification front' which advances steadily through the bone matrix as it is formed. During active bone formation there is a thin layer of uncalcified matrix (an osteoid seam) on top of the calcification front (Fig. 7.1). When bone formation stops the matrix becomes fully calcified. If calcification is impeded the front moves more slowly so that the osteoid seams are wider than normal but the centres of the trabeculae are calcified normally. Bone is being destroyed and reformed continuously. The exact role of the bone cells is still uncertain but *osteoblasts* seem to make collagen and *osteoclasts* destroy bone with matrix and bone crystals dissolving simultaneously. The skeleton of a young adult contains about 1 kg of calcium but only about 0.1% is in equilibrium with body fluids and the rest is accessible only by bone remodelling over years.

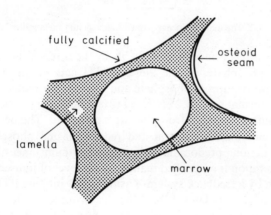

Fig. 7.1. Structure of normal cancellous bone. Shaded area is calcified.

PARATHYROID GLANDS

Anatomy

The parathyroid glands are thin reddish-brown spindles about 5 mm long but variable in size and shape. Usually there are two glands on each side, one high and one low, lying behind and medial to the lateral lobes of the thyroid and close to the trachea but they may be anywhere from the jaw to the thymus and sometimes within the thyroid gland.

Chapter 7

Physiology

Parathyroid hormone (PTH) is a straight chain polypeptide containing eighty-four aminoacids. The biological activity resides mainly in the 1–29 amino terminal acids. PTH can be measured in human plasma by radioimmunoassay. The metabolism of calcium and phosphate and the maintenance of the skeleton is under the close control of PTH (Fig. 7.2).

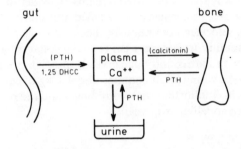

Fig. 7.2. The main influences controlling calcium metabolism.

On bone its effect is mediated probably by the osteoclasts to liberate calcium and phosphate. In the kidney, PTH acts on the tubule to reduce the reabsorption of phosphate and increase the reabsorption of calcium. The formation of 1,25 (OH_2) D_3 (see below) is accelerated by PTH so calcium absorption from the gut is enhanced. The net effect of PTH is to raise plasma calcium and reduce plasma phosphate but which of its actions predominates in various circumstances is uncertain. PTH secretion is controlled mainly by the level of ionised calcium in the plasma by a feedback system—rising Ca^{++} inhibits PTH release and falling Ca^{++} stimulates it. No other factor directly affecting PTH release has been discovered but the occurrence of parathyroid hyperplasia in some patients with primary hyperparathyroidism and raised plasma calcium suggests that another factor might exist. Also, in some individuals a normal parathyroid response to a fall in plasma calcium does not occur, implying the lack of some essential factor.

CALCITONIN

This is a second calcium controlling hormone. It is secreted by the parafollicular cells of the thyroid. It is a polypeptide with thirty-two aminoacids and a 1–7 disulphide bridge at the carboxyl end. It acts more quickly than PTH. It depresses osteoclast function and tends to lower plasma calcium but its role in physiology is uncertain. Medullary carcinomas of the thyroid secrete large amounts of calcitonin and a high blood level provides a useful diagnostic test, but there is no apparent disturbance of calcium metabolism. Therapeutic injections of calcitonin may be used in treating Paget's disease of bone.

VITAMIN D

'Vitamin D' is now appreciated as a complex hormonal system with nutritional implications. In the skin the action of the shorter wave length component of ultraviolet light converts 7-dehydrocholesterol to pre-cholecalciferol which isomerises slowly to cholecalciferol or Vitamin D_3 (Fig. 7.3).

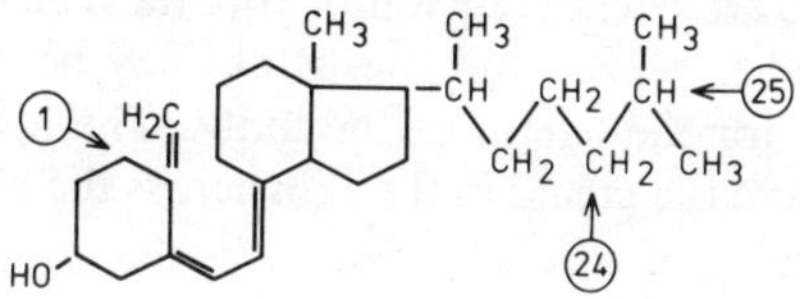

FIG. 7.3. Cholecalciferol or Vitamin D_3. The carbon positions C-1, C-24 and C-25 are indicated.

The vitamin of the diet and that used in therapy is *ergocalciferol* or Vitamin D_2. In the liver D_2 and D_3 are hydroxylated at the '25' position to form e.g. 25 hydroxycholecalciferol (25–OH D_3). In the kidney there is a further hydroxylation at the '1' position. This is accelerated by PTH and the product 1,25 $(OH)_2$ D_3 (sometimes written as '1,25 DHCC') is the effective and highly potent hormone. The D_2 and D_3 derivatives are equally active. The principal roles of 1,25 DHCC are to promote the absorption of calcium from the gut and the calcification of bone matrix. In the kidney 24,25 (OH_2) D_3 may be formed also but it is relatively inert. The differential hydroxylation at the C-1 or C-24 position may constitute a control system.

METABOLIC BONE DISEASE

This term indicates a bone disease which is generalised, although not always uniform, in contradistinction to localised bone disease such as primary or secondary tumours and Paget's disease. Many causes and related factors are known but there are only three main forms.

Osteoporosis

This is by far the commonest generalised disease of bone. There is a reduction in bone mass due to an imbalance between the rate of bone formation and resorption. The remaining bone is normal both histologically and biochemically. Because of this apparent normality and because the condition arises from a wasting of the bone there is no exact division between the normal and osteoporotic skeleton.

Clinical features

There is no specific change in general health and the bone in itself is painless. Nevertheless, pain is a principal symptom because osteoporotic bone is brittle and distortion or fracture of bone is common in this condition. Backache is frequent due to vertebral body collapse or associated degenerative arthritis; many patients sustain fractures of ribs or long bones after relatively minor trauma. The physical signs are loss of height and kyphosis and the trunk may be obviously shorter than appropriate for the length of the limbs. The lower ribs meet the iliac crests and there is a crease in the skin across the upper abdomen.

Causes

A slowly progressive osteoporosis is a normal feature of ageing. In people in their 70's the skeleton has on average only half the bulk of that in young people. Because osteoporosis appears to be part of the normal ageing process it is debatable whether it should be regarded as a disease. Perhaps persons with particularly marked and symptomatic osteoporosis are only the extreme end of a normal distribution curve.

Menopause. Skeletal bulk is maintained until the menopause but afterwards skeletal wasting begins due, presumably, to the withdrawal of oestrogen. As in old age the process is much more marked in some persons than others.

Immobilisation. Normal stress on bone is necessary for the maintenance of normal structure. Local or general inactivity from any cause leads to local or general bone wasting respectively.

Rheumatoid arthritis. A local osteoporosis by affected joints is characteristic but a general osteoporosis is common, due perhaps to immobilisation and/or corticosteroids (see below).

Endocrine disorders. Changes in endocrine function can cause osteoporosis, particularly increased glucocorticoid action, spontaneously in Cushing's syndrome or from the administration of corticosteroids, natural or synthetic (see Chapter 8). Osteoporosis may occur in hyperthyroidism and sex hormone deficiency (see appropriate section).

Others. Osteoporosis may occur in severe and prolonged malnutrition. In some patients no cause can be found ('idiopathic osteoporosis'). Osteogenesis imperfecta is an inherited disorder which usually presents with multiple fractures in early life but in adults is indistinguishable from idiopathic osteoporosis. There may be an unusual blue appearance of the sclerae due to a defect of collagen formation which presumably is also the cause of the bone condition.

Diagnosis

The biochemical findings are essentially normal. If the osteoporosis is proceeding rapidly the urine calcium may rise. Radiology shows diminished bone density but this is a crude index and perhaps as much as 50% of the skeletal mass has to be lost before a definite change is seen. More specifically, the cortex of the bone is thinned and the trabecula markings attenuated. The collapse of the vertebral bodies with consequent 'wedging' is characteristic, usually in the zone D6 to L2 but sometimes elsewhere. Vertebral collapse from metastatic disease or tuberculosis can usually be identified by the presence of adjacent bone destruction, particularly in the neural arches. Sometimes, vertebral discs herniate into the vertebral bodies causing the so-called 'cod-fish' appearance but this is uncommon and is more likely to indicate osteomalacia.

Treatment

The management of osteoporosis is unsatisfactory. Fractures of long bones unite normally and vertebral collapse becomes painless after a few weeks. Spinal supports may relieve the pain of associated osteoarthritis but generally are of little use. The maintenance of normal physical activity and a normal mixed diet are probably helpful. Unless a specific cause can be removed no treatment will lead to restoration of normal bone and the best that can be hoped for is that the process can be arrested or slowed down. It has been claimed that small doses of calciferol are helpful but this is not generally accepted. Oestrogens and androgens are widely used and there is evidence that oestrogens in the post-menopausal woman will arrest osteoporosis but the treatment may carry some risk of thrombosis and uterine carcinogenesis. Intermittent therapy and combination with a progestogen is thought to be safer. Androgens can be used in men, probably with similar benefit. The so-called non-virilising androgens (see Chapter 9) have been recommended for this purpose.

Prognosis
The common form of post-menopausal or senile osteoporosis is slowly progressive but does not shorten life except by increasing the risk of fractures. Senile osteoporosis and its consequences pose a serious public health problem in the UK and effective preventive measures are not currently available.

Osteomalacia and rickets

These names refer to the same condition but 'rickets' is used to label the condition in children while 'osteomalacia' is used usually in respect of adults and also the histological appearances (see 'Pathology', below).

Clinical features

Children. This condition virtually disappeared in the UK during and after the Second World War because of an extensive public health campaign to encourage the use of cheap vitamin D supplements in childhood and infant feeding. Recently the condition has reappeared particularly among children of Asian racial origin. The aetiology is obscure and not now related to neglect (see below). The child is likely to be generally unwell, fails to thrive and grows slowly. The older child complains of pain in the joints and legs. In the florid case the joints (particularly the wrists and costo-chondral joints) are swollen and skeletal deformities may occur. A primary condition (e.g. coeliac disease or renal failure) may be present.

Adult. The predominant complaint is of pain which may be related to the joints, or to the long bones, particularly in the legs. Bony tenderness may be present. The patients often have a characteristic 'waddling' gait which is due partly to pain but partly also to proximal muscle weakness due to vitamin D deficiency.

In non-Asian Caucasians in the UK osteomalacia is likely to be secondary to another disease such as intestinal malabsorption (particularly adult coeliac disease) or chronic renal failure. The vitamin D deficiency may be caused by long-term anticonvulsant therapy. It may be found in elderly persons, particularly women, taking restricted diets.

In women of Asian racial origin osteomalacia is common particularly during pregnancy.

Pathology
The level of calcium in the plasma tends to fall with consequent secondary hyperparathyroidism causing a reduction in plasma phosphate and an increase in plasma alkaline phosphatase. In a few patients, for no apparent reason, the expected parathyroid response does not take place, the plasma calcium falls further and tetany may occur. Matrix formation in the bone is normal but calcification is delayed so that the osteoid seams are wider and more extensive than normal. In children, the epiphyseal plates are deranged in a complex but characteristic fashion.

Aetiology
The cause of the rickets in Asians living in the UK is uncertain. Three theories are current: (i) lack of sunlight action due to climate, skin pigment, traditional clothing and a tendency for the young women to stay indoors, (ii) diet, which may depend heavily on rice, clarified butter and be largely or wholly vegetarian, (iii) the use of 'Chuppatis' which are lightly cooked from unleavened flour and therefore contain large amounts of phytate which may reduce calcium absorption. All the theories are plausible but conclusive evidence is lacking.

Diagnosis
Initial suspicion is circumstantial depending on ethnic group, social circumstances and predisposing disease. The full clinical picture is diagnostic but minor forms with pain and abnormal gait are more common. Radiographs are often normal but in the more severe case the typical appearance of Looser's zones (pseudo fractures or Milkman's fractures) are seen. These are narrow bands of translucency, like incomplete fractures, most commonly in the pubic ramus, edge of scapula, clavicle, rib and neck of femur. In children typical changes are present in the epiphyseal plates. Occasionally 'cod-fish' vertebrae are seen. Probably the best single biochemical index is a raised plasma bone alkaline phosphatase but this is an unreliable guide in the adolescent because the level is usually raised during puberty. The level of plasma calcium is depressed but often only slightly. It seems that the secondary hyperparathyroidism which results prevents a further fall in calcium but also leads to the typical depression of plasma phosphate. The urine calcium is an unreliable guide. Biochemical evidence of an underlying cause, e.g. renal tubular failure or intestinal malabsorption, may be present.

Treatment
In the nutritional form, oral calciferol supplements are curative.

In theory, only physiological quantities, e.g. 25 mg (1000 units) per day should suffice but in practice 1.25 mg (50000 units) per day for a short time is more certain, followed by a maintenance supplement of 25 mg or so per day. In secondary forms larger doses for longer periods may be needed with other supplements depending on circumstances.

Prognosis
Pain should be relieved in a few weeks and radiological healing should be complete in a few months. Relapse is common if supplements are not maintained.

Hyperparathyroid bone disease (Osteitis fibrosa)

This is now a relatively uncommon feature of primary hyperparathyroidism (see below). In the florid example, decalcified bone sections show an increased number of osteoclasts, often multinucleate, clustering along the surface of trabeculae made irregular by increased and disorganised bone destruction. The marrow is infiltrated by fibrous tissue. Whole bone sections show slight widening and extension of the osteoid seams, even in primary hyperparathyroidism with a raised plasma calcium. In the secondary form, the osteoid seams are more marked.

Radiologically, there is usually some demineralisation but this is slight and occasionally bone density is increased. The characteristic appearance is of subperiosteal erosions which are most readily seen in the phalanges. The bone architecture seems blurred, as if it were out of focus, particularly in the lateral skull film. There may be cysts several centimetres across in the long bones. Treatment is that of hyperparathyroidism.

Renal osteodystrophy

This term is applied to the bone disease which occurs commonly in chronic uraemia and in patients on prolonged haemodialysis. It is not a specific condition but consists of a mixture of the changes of osteomalacia and secondary hyperparathyroidism. In individual patients, different features predominate, depending perhaps on the degree of parathyroid response. Sometimes there is a marked increase in bone density (*osteosclerosis*) for unknown reasons. It may show in a widening of the vertebral plates producing the appearance of the so-called 'rugger jersey' spine. Treatment may be difficult. 1,25 DHCC is useful to raise the plasma calcium but removal of hypertrophied parathyroid glands may be necessary.

HYPERCALCAEMIA

Clinical features
The normal level of total plasma calcium is 2.3–2.6 mmol/l. Even slight variations above that range are significant if persistent. For best reliability blood should be drawn with the patient fasting and without venous stasis.

Slight hypercalcaemia, i.e. up to 3.0 mmol/l is symptomless and even levels of 3.5 mmol/l do not necessarily cause symptoms. At higher levels symptoms appear but are non-specific. The most common ones are muscle weakness, anorexia and nausea, constipation and weight loss. Polyuria and polydipsia may be marked and mental changes occur ranging from apathy to dementia.

The only specific physical signs are in the eyes where band keratitis (deposits of calcium in the edge of the cornea) and calcium deposits in the conjunctivae may occur. The latter appear as tiny glistening papules in the palpebral fissure. The ECG shows shortening of the Q–T interval.

Differential diagnosis
Measurement of urine calcium is not helpful in differential diagnosis. Plasma phosphate may be misleading and the various phosphate clearance calculations are little better. Usually, the associated circumstances, hormone assays and bone radiology will establish the cause.

Relatively common causes	Uncommon causes
Hyperparathyroidism	Addison's disease
Malignant disease, with or without bony metastases	Hypercalcaemia of infancy
Vitamin D intoxication	Hypophosphatasia
Hyperthyroidism	Acute osteoporosis of disuse
Sarcoidosis	Milk–alkali syndrome

Treatment
Mild hypercalcaemia calls for no treatment until investigation has led to a definitive diagnosis and treatment of the primary condition. Immediate treatment of severe symptomatic hypercalcaemia is by:
1. Replacement of water and salt deficiency.

2. Corticosteroids are helpful in malignant disease, sarcoidosis and vitamin D intoxication.
3. Phosphate. This may be given orally as sodium phosphate in a dose of 500 mg elemental phosphorus 2–6 times daily. This is usually rapidly effective and the results persist for several days. Long-term use may cause soft-tissue calcification.
4. Calcitonin may be effective.
5. Mithramycin.

HYPOCALCAEMIA

Clinical features
Minor degrees of hypocalcaemia (e.g. down to 2.0 mmol/l) are symptomless. Lower levels produce paraesthesiae around the mouth and of the extremities, going on to muscle cramps, tetany (painful flexor spasms) and convulsions. Longstanding hypocalcaemia is usually less obvious and may present with lethargy and cramps, mental symptoms with depression or psychosis, or epilepsy alone.

The two cardinal clinical tests of hypocalcaemia are designed to reveal latent tetany.

Chvostek's sign consists of observing a contraction of the facial muscles at the corner of the mouth and in the cheeks in response to a tap over the branches of the facial nerve as they emerge from the anterior border of the parotid gland on that side. Some movement can be seen in many normal persons but a brisk contraction, particularly if it changes with time, is significant.

Trousseau's sign is elicited by inflating a sphygmomanometer cuff on the upper arm until the systolic pressure is exceeded; this pressure is then maintained. Muscle spasm in the forearm producing the 'main d'accoucheur' appearance, as in tetany, does not occur in normal persons in less than three minutes.

Differential diagnosis
Lack of vitamin D	Nutritional
Renal tubular defects	Malabsorption
Hypoparathyroidism	Uraemia

A reduction in plasma calcium from any cause will usually result in a secondary hyperparathyroidism so the features of that (low plasma phosphate and raised alkaline phosphatase) are not helpful in differential diagnosis. In hypoparathyroidism plasma phosphate tends to rise while PTH is low, but this may only indicate a failure of parathyroid response in a patient with hypocalcaemia from another cause.

Treatment
Emergency treatment is by slow intravenous injection of calcium gluconate 10% in water. The dose is 1–2 g, i.e. 10–20 ml. This may be repeated as necessary or given by a slow intravenous infusion diluted in saline. There is a serious *danger of overdosage* which may cause cardiac arrest. Oral calcium supplements are relatively ineffective and large numbers of tablets may be needed. The proprietary effervescent tablets are better and provide 400 mg calcium each. A syrup is available. For long-term treatment oral calciferol is needed. The dose is dependent on circumstances and is discussed below (see hypoparathyroidism). There is rarely any need for calciferol injections.

HYPERPARATHYROIDISM

Primary

This is caused by excessive autonomous release of PTH.

Clinical features
Women are affected about four times as frequently as men, usually in middle or later life. It is now appreciated as a relatively common condition with an *annual* incidence of about 30 per 100000 people. The advent of biochemical screening has altered the usual clinical picture. The natural history of the condition covers many years but it is not known why its course varies so much in different individuals.

About half the patients are asymptomatic at diagnosis, the plasma calcium having been measured during screening or the investigation of other diseases. Most of the remainder present with renal calculi but some patients have symptoms directly caused by hypercalcaemia—these include tiredness, weakness (particularly of proximal muscles), anorexia, weight loss, thirst, polyuria, constipation and dementia. Rarely, peptic ulceration and pancreatitis may occur. Few patients present with bone disease. Previous irradiation of the neck may be a predisposing factor.

Physical examination is not specific. A considerable proportion of the patients have hypertension and the incidence of diabetes is higher than would be expected by chance. Corneal calcification (see above under 'Hypercalcaemia') may be seen and bony deformities may be present. It is most unusual for a parathyroid adenoma to be palpable in the neck.

Pathology

Usually there is a small benign adenoma of one parathyroid gland and the other glands are atrophied. Rarely the tumour is a carcinoma. In 10–20% of patients some or all of the glands are hypertrophied. Histologically, the adenomas usually contain 'chief' cells while 'water clear' cells are present in the hyperplastic glands, but often the picture is mixed and hyperplasia cannot always be differentiated from adenoma. Thus there is uncertainty as to whether multiple adenomas ever occur or whether they are really hyperplastic glands. Parathyroid adenoma may be part of a multiple endocrine adenomatosis (see Chapter 13).

Renal damage is common. There may be changes in tubular function, which are usually reversible, but nephrocalcinosis and permanent renal damage may occur. The high urine calcium promotes the formation of renal calculi.

Bone disease is probably always present but it is usually slight and then it can be detected only by special methods. The features are described above.

Diagnosis

Except where typical radiological changes are present the diagnosis is likely to be suspected from clinical features but always requires biochemical confirmation. The plasma calcium is the key to the diagnosis—fasting blood should be drawn without venous stasis. A persistently raised value, i.e. more than 2.6 mmol/l is significant but sometimes the level fluctuates and may be normal on occasions or even for long periods. Repeated estimations over several months are most helpful and permit diagnosis by exclusion because during that time it can be determined that malignant disease, sarcoidosis and calciferol intoxication are not present. The level of plasma proteins may be important; mild hypercalcaemia may be caused by raised proteins or masked by low proteins. Conversion factors may be applied but are rarely needed. The plasma PTH may be helpful, particularly if it is inappropriately high in relation to the plasma calcium but not infrequently the level is within the normal range.

A low plasma phosphate (i.e. below 0.8 mmol/l) would be expected but often the level is normal, particularly if renal failure is present. The plasma alkaline phosphatase is usually normal unless obvious bone disease is present. The urinary calcium excretion is usually high but is influenced by so many factors, particularly dietary intake and renal function, that no reliance can be placed on it.

The hydrocortisone suppression test involves giving 40 mg hydrocortisone thrice daily by mouth for ten days and observing the effect on the plasma calcium. In hyperparathyroidism there is little or no effect, whereas other forms of hypercalcaemia should respond with a fall in calcium. The test is not always reliable and equivocal results are common.

Treatment

An increasing number of patients with no symptoms or with only trivial or intermittent complaints are being found to have hyperparathyroidism. This is forcing the consideration of conservative treatment and some patients are now managed in this way. There is doubt about the safety of doing so and some claim that the danger of progressive insidious renal damage still makes surgery mandatory. However, some patients seem to do well and avoid the inconvenience, discomfort, danger and scars of surgery for many years. Regular supervision with review of plasma calcium and renal function is essential.

Patients who have had a renal calculus are usually considered to be at risk and surgery is advised, but, even in these patients, if surgery is refused, it may be many years before a further stone appears. Apart from conservative management medical treatment is of little help. Oestrogen has been advised for post-menopausal women but seems to have little effect. Sodium phosphate may be used to lower the plasma calcium but this treatment carries a risk of ectopic calcification and is only suitable for long-term use as a last resort.

The definitive treatment is surgical. The operation may be tedious and difficult if the tumour is small. Preoperative localisation of the tumour has been unreliable but measuring PTH in blood samples from veins draining the neck may identify the site of excess production. Ideally the surgeon should identify and confirm by frozen section all the glands as well as removing the tumour. If hyperplasia is present only a fragment of one gland is left in place. If a tumour cannot be located in the neck the upper mediastinum is explored and occasionally a sternotomy is necessary. Exploration destroys the tissue planes and a second operation is much more difficult; it is of prime importance that the first operation is conclusive. For patients without bone disease no preoperative preparation is needed and the plasma calcium need not be lowered unless it is so high that the patient is symptomatic. Slight to moderate hypercalcaemia is not an anaesthetic hazard. In patients with bone disease, calciferol or its metabolites may be given to reduce the later skeletal avidity for calcium. Post-operatively, the patient must be examined for latent tetany and the plasma calcium measured frequently. A fall in plasma calcium may occur within twelve hours but more commonly over several days. A good fall to below normal is gratifying as it indicates successful surgery but a further fall must be prevented by oral or intravenous calcium and calciferol as necessary (see treatment of hypoparathyroidism, below).

Long-term follow up to detect recurrence is desirable. After successful surgery the bones should heal completely and life expectancy be normal but hypertension and renal damage may persist and mar the outcome.

Secondary

This occurs when the parathyroids are stimulated to release excessive PTH by a persistently low level of plasma calcium from any cause.

Clinical features

The presentation is dominated by the underlying disease. The secondary hyperparathyroidism is usually a biochemical finding but bone X-rays may show features similar to those of primary hyperparathyroidism in addition to demineralisation and pseudo-fractures (see above).

Pathology and diagnosis

There is a slight to moderate enlargement of all the parathyroid glands with variable histological appearances. It is curious that in some patients, particularly those with uraemia, a normal parathyroid response does not occur, the plasma calcium falls markedly and tetany may recur. With the normal parathyroid response the plasma calcium is maintained close to or just within the normal range and tetany is rare.

The diagnosis is made by a raised plasma bone alkaline phosphatase with or without typical bone X-rays, in the presence of a reduced or low normal plasma calcium. Urine calcium is low and plasma phosphate also, except in uraemia. The differentiation between primary and secondary hyperparathyroidism can nearly always be made by the level of the plasma calcium but difficulties can arise— the primary disease may be normocalcaemic and the secondary form produce a raised calcium apparently contrary to physiological principles.

Treatment

This consists of the management of the primary disease with attempts to raise the plasma calcium by calcium supplements and/or calciferol. If the primary disease is intractable parathyroidectomy may be considered to relieve crippling bone disease.

'Tertiary' hyperparathyroidism

This term is applied to a situation in which apparently primary hyperparathyroidism with a tumour is found in a patient who was known to have prolonged hypocalcaemia previously. It is supposed that in response to this there was parathyroid hyperplasia (secondary hyperparathyroidism) and then an autonomous adenoma developed in a hyperplastic gland. In patients presenting for the first time with chronic uraemia and hypercalcaemia the differentiation of primary and tertiary hyperparathyroidism cannot be made.

HYPOPARATHYROIDISM

Clinical features

The symptoms are mostly those of hypocalcaemia (see above), particularly epilepsy. In the congenital form there may be calcification of the basal ganglia and mental retardation. Later, the fingernails become brittle and monilial infection of the nails and skin occur. Cataracts are common. The physical signs are of latent tetany (see above). Compensation for the lack of PTH may be quite good and the patient live a comparatively normal life for years before the diagnosis is made.

Aetiology and pathology

Surgical. By far the commonest cause of hypoparathyroidism is damage to or removal of the parathyroid glands during surgery to the thyroid or larynx. The condition may be temporary, perhaps due to interruption of blood supply, or permanent.

Idiopathic. This is a rare disease, due perhaps to an autoimmune process, whereby the parathyroid glands are destroyed, usually early in life. There is no specific pathology except the absence of the parathyroid glands.

Diagnosis

This is based on finding a persistently low level of plasma calcium coupled with a failure of parathyroid response as indicated by a normal or raised plasma phosphate and a normal alkaline phosphatase. The absence of a raised level of plasma PTH is important also. Finding the other pathological features mentioned above may be helpful. There are no consistent changes in the skeleton.

Treatment
Immediate treatment is by intravenous or oral calcium (see above) but long-term treatment depends on vitamin D to enhance calcium absorption from the gut and thus maintain the plasma level. A relatively large dose of calciferol is required presumably to overcome the low production rate of 1,25 DHCC due to the lack of PTH. It is reasonable to start with 2.5 mg (100,000 units) of calciferol a day but the usual maintenance dose is between 1.25 and 2.5 mg/d and fine adjustment of dose may be needed. The standard tablets are of 1.25 mg and 0.25 mg so considerable care in prescribing and patient compliance are needed. The effect is slowly cumulative, so that there may be long-term trends in the level of plasma calcium; in practice it is unsatisfactory to change the dose more frequently than once a week. Regular measurements of plasma calcium are essential particularly in the early stages; it is easy to produce hypercalcaemia even within the normal therapeutic range. It is best to aim at maintaining the plasma calcium towards the lower limit of normal. The requirements for calciferol may change so long-term follow up is necessary. If the patient is taking a relatively normal diet oral calcium supplements are of little help in treatment and are so tedious to take that overall compliance in therapy may be reduced but milk may be a useful supplement as each 500 ml contains about 600 mg of calcium. Synthetic 1,25 DHCC and 1αHCC are available. The latter is equally effective as the C-25 hydroxylation takes place readily in the liver. Their effect is fully comparable with calciferol and their action is somewhat faster. The doses are much lower (1 to 3 mg/d) as there is no need to overcome the difficulty with the C-1 hydroxylation. The use of these more expensive compounds is justified in the treatment of renal osteodystrophy but in other patients their advantage over calciferol is unproved.

Prognosis
If the plasma calcium can be maintained in the normal range the outlook is good and normal pregnancy is possible.

PSEUDO-HYPOPARATHYROIDISM

In this very rare condition some or all of the biochemical features of hypoparathyroidism occur in the presence of normal or raised levels of PTH due, presumably, to an insensitivity of the tissues to the hormone. Several types have been described. The condition can be diagnosed by demonstrating a failure of renal response to injected parathyroid hormone.

FURTHER READING

BRESLAU N.A. & PAK C.Y.C. (1979). Hypoparathyroidism. *Metabolism*, **28**, 1261.

GRIMELIUS L. *et al* (1979). Controversies in the treatment of hyperparathyroidism. *Acta Chirurgica Scandinavica*, **145**, 355.

JUAN D. (1979). Hypocalcemia. *Archives of Internal Medicine*, **139**, 1166.

LEWIN I.G. *et al* (1978). Studies of hypoparathyroidism and pseudohypoparathyroidism. *Quarterly Journal of Medicine*, **47**, 533.

SCHNEIDER A.B. & SHERWOOD L.M. (1975). Pathogenesis and management of hypoparathyroidism and other hypocalcemic disorders. *Metabolism*, **24**, 871.

SCHOLZ D.A. *et al* (1978). Primary hyperparathyroidism with multiple parathyroid gland involvement. *Mayo Clinic Proceedings*, **53**, 792.

STANBURY S.W. (1981). Vitamin D: metamorphosis from nutrient to hormonal system. *Proceedings of the Nutrition Society*, **40**, 179.

WELLS S.A.J. *et al* (1980). Primary hyperparathyroidism. *Current Problems in Surgery*, **17**, 398.

Chapter 8
Pituitary and Hypothalamus

ANATOMY

Hypothalmic–pituitary unit

The hypothalamus is a somewhat arbitrarily defined anatomical zone which includes the floor of the third ventricle, the median eminence and some adjacent structures beneath the thalamus. The endocrine function of the areas of the hypothalamus in man is poorly defined. Veins from the median eminence combine to form the plexus of portal veins in the pituitary stalk which provides nearly all the blood supply to the anterior pituitary gland (adenohypophysis). This part has virtually no neural connections. The supra-optic and paraventricular nuclei have large nerve tracts through the stalk to the posterior pituitary gland (neurohypophysis) which has a normal arterial blood supply. There is a small intermediate part of the pituitary which is of doubtful significance in man.

The pituitary gland in adults weighs about 0.5 g and lies in a depression in the sphenoid bone called the pituitary fossa or sella turcica. The pituitary gland has no capsule and is continuous with the adjacent structures including the diaphragma sellae above and the medial walls of the cavernous venous sinuses on either side.

The anterior pituitary comprises a mixture of different types of cell, each forming a largely independent system. The sources of most of the pituitary hormones can be recognised by special histologic techniques but the older classifications based on simple staining reactions are inadequate. In particular, chromophobe cells may secrete growth hormone or prolactin. The distribution of cells in the anterior pituitary is not random. There are relatively more cells secreting growth hormone and prolactin at the sides of the gland with more cells secreting thyrotrophin and corticotrophin in the centre. Gonadotrophin secreting cells are distributed throughout.

PHYSIOLOGY

Hypothalamic hormones

These are mostly short-chain polypeptides and are synthesised in the hypothalamus, stored in the median eminence and then released to pass down the portal venous system to the sinusoids of the anterior pituitary where they control—by stimulation or inhibition—the release of the anterior pituitary hormones. The hypothalmic hormones recognised so far are:

Releasing hormones
1. Thyrotrophin releasing hormone (TRH) is a tripeptide which is available for clinical use. It is also a potent releasing hormone for prolactin.
2. Luteinising hormone/follicle stimulating hormone releasing hormone (LH/FSH–RH or LHRH) is a decapeptide which releases both gonadotrophins.

3. *Corticotrophin releasing hormone* (CRH; a more complex peptide) (Other releasing hormones have been postulated).

Inhibitory hormones
1. *Growth hormone release inhibiting hormone* (somatostatin).
2. *Prolactin release inhibiting hormone* (dopamine).

With one exception (somatostatin) the hypothalamic hormones appear to have actions limited to the appropriate cells of the anterior pituitary although they may have actions within the brain. Somatostatin has been located in tissues other than the hypothalamus, e.g. the pancreatic islets. When given parenterally it blocks the effect of TRH and suppresses the release of growth hormone, prolactin, insulin and glucagon. The physiological role of this extraordinary substance is uncertain.

Anterior pituitary hormones

The anterior pituitary in man secretes six or seven peptide hormones.

Thyroid stimulating hormone (TSH or thyrotrophin)
This is a glycoprotein which consists of two polypeptide chains, α and β. The α chain is the same in the other two glycoprotein pituitary hormones, LH, and FSH (see below) and the biological activity resides in the β chain. TSH effects only the thyroid gland, having a stimulating effect on many of its activities including iodide uptake, hormone synthesis, thyroglobulin synthesis and hormone release. TSH increases the height of the follicle epithelium, the size of the gland and its vascularity.

Luteinising hormone (LH; or interstitial cell stimulating hormone: ICSH).
This hormone specifically stimulates the formation and secretion of the corpus luteum, and acts also with FSH (see below) to promote the development of the follicle and cause ovulation. LH stimulates the Leydig cells in the testis to synthesise and secrete testosterone.

Follicle stimulating hormone (FSH)
This stimulates the development of the follicle in the ovary. In the testis FSH stimulates the germinal epithelium of the testicular tubules causing spermatogenesis.

(LH and FSH are both glycoproteins with an α and β chain, the latter carrying the biological activity.)

Adrenocorticotrophin (ACTH or corticotrophin)
This is a 39 amino acid polypeptide in which the biological activity depends on the segment 1 to 24 while the segment 25 to 33 contains the species differences and immunological specificity (Fig. 8.1) (see lipotrophin below).

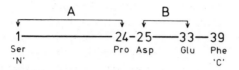

FIG. 8.1. The structure of corticotrophin. The 'N' and 'C' terminals are indicated. Bracket 'A' indicates the area in which the biological activity is located and bracket 'B' the area of species specificity Ser = serine, Pro = proline, Asp = aspartic acid, Glu = glutamic acid, Phe = phenylalanine.

ACTH stimulates the growth of the adrenal cortex and the conversion of cholesterol to pregnenolone causing increased steroidogenesis. ACTH also has extra-adrenal affects of doubtful physiological significance in man.

Growth hormone (GH or somatotrophin)
This is a 191 amino acid polypeptide which is similar to prolactin. It is the only anterior pituitary hormone with physiological effects on many tissues. The mode of action of GH is uncertain but it is likely that it acts on the liver to produce *somatomedins* (or sulfation factor). These are relatively simple peptides which induce growth promoting activities in many tissues. There are effects also on carbohydrate and fat metabolism but nevertheless GH is not essential for normal health in the adult.

Prolactin (PRL)
The primary role of this hormone is milk production but it has important influences on sexual function and fertility.

Lipotrophins
α lipotrophin with 58 amino acids and ß lipotrophin with 91 amino acids are two large polypeptides released from the ACTH secreting cells. The functions of the lipotrophins themselves are uncertain but β lipotrophin contains within its peptide chain the amino acid sequences of β endorphin, melanocyte stimulating hormone (β MSH) and ACTH. The significance of this and the interrelationship of the compounds is not known.

Posterior pituitary hormones

There are two very similar octapeptide posterior pituitary hormones, *vasopressin* (anti-diuretic hormone or ADH) and *oxytocin* (Fig. 8.2).

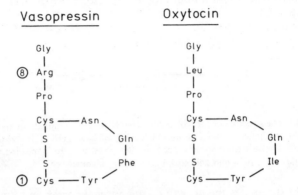

FIG. 8.2. The structures of vasopressin and oxytocin. Gly = glycine, Arg = arginine, Pro = proline, Cys = cysteine, Asn = asparagine, Tyr = tyrosine, Leu = leucine, Ile = isoleucine, Phe = phenylalanine, Gln = glutamine. Lysine vasopressin has lysine instead of arginine. Desmopressin is 1-desamino 8-D-arginine vasopressin.

These substances are synthesised in the hypothalamic nuclei connected to the neuro-hypophysis. The hormones are bound by the protein neurophysin(s) and pass along the axons of the neurohypophyseal tract in secondary granules and accumulate in the posterior pituitary from which they are released. Vasopressin in large doses can cause smooth muscle contraction and increase blood pressure (hence its name) but its only physiological action is on the nephron. It has an anti-diuretic affect by increasing the permeability to water of the distal tubule and collecting duct thus increasing the concentration and reducing the volume of the urine. Oxytocin acts on the breast to cause milk ejection and also contracts the myometrium but despite these apparently important functions its physiological role in man is uncertain.

Control of anterior pituitary function

The secretion of the various hormones is controlled by complex processes which are mostly, but not entirely, independent. For three hormones a known feed-back exists (Fig. 8.3), in that the product of the endocrine end organ modulates the secretion of the stimulating substance. It is not clear whether the 'peripheral' hormones act by suppressing the release of the hypothalamic hormones or reducing the sensitivity of the pituitary cells to the hypothalamic hormones. Many drugs, biochemical changes and emotional factors can affect the secretion of pituitary hormones. It is presumed that they act via the hypothalamus but some of the effects may be directly on the pituitary. The biological rhythms of pituitary hormone release are presumably mediated via the hypothalamus but the site of generation of the rhythms is uncertain.

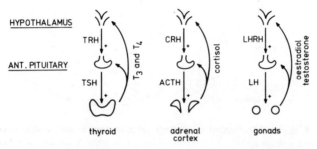

FIG. 8.3. The hypothalamic-anterior pituitary control 'loops' for thyroid, adrenal cortex and sex hormones.

TSH
The release of TSH is stimulated by TRH but little is known about the control of TRH secretion—it seems little affected by brain activity. Plasma levels of free T_3 and T_4 modulate the secretion of TSH, and high levels of T_3 and T_4 suppress the responsiveness of the pituitary to exogenous TRH.

ACTH
The release of ACTH is stimulated by CRH. Although ACTH stimulates the production of various steroids from the adrenal cortex it is only cortisol (and the synthetic corticosteroids) which modulate the secretion of ACTH. The secretion of ACTH has a marked diurnal rhythm which controls the diurnal rhythm of plasma cortisol. ACTH secretion is stimulated by many different kinds of 'stress' but particularly emotional stress and fear, physical injury such as surgery or infection and chemical changes such as hypoglycaemia. Secretion can be suppressed by cyproheptadine.

LH
Secretion is stimulated by LHRH and modulated by oestradiol, testosterone and many synthetic analogues. There is some diurnal fluctu-

ation of LH release but a much more marked variation during the menstrual cycle, particularly the sudden mid-cycle peak. This seems to be due to an increase in sensitivity of the pituitary to LHRH caused by oestrogen. Emotional factors and changes in body weight (probably interrelated) can affect LH release and therefore ovulation.

For the other three anterior pituitary hormones the control of secretion is more complex and less well-understood (Fig. 8.4).

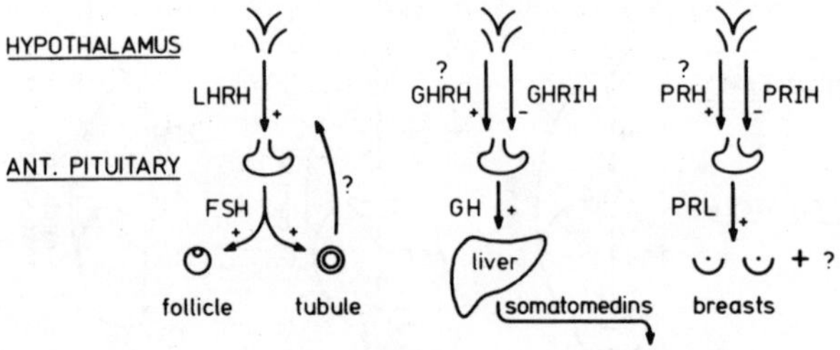

FIG. 8.4. Hypothalmic-anterior pituitary relationships in which the control 'loops' are unknown.

FSH

The release of FSH is stimulated by LHRH. At times, FSH and LH are released independently but how is unknown. The feed-back control of FSH is disputed—secretion can be suppressed by oestradiol or testosterone but on the other hand FSH secretion is increased if the seminiferous epithelium is destroyed, despite normal levels of testosterone. An inhibitor of FSH secretion called 'inhibin' from the seminiferous epithelium has been proposed but not identified.

GH

The release of GH is markedly episodic. It is stimulated by sleep, stress such as exercise or hypoglycaemia and the intake of amino acids, particularly arginine. No feed-back system for GH is known except perhaps via glucose levels.

PRL

Secretion probably takes place spontaneously and control is exercised by varying degrees of inhibition depending on dopamine from the hypothalamus. There is a marked diurnal rhythm with a peak in the early hours of the morning in non-pregnant women and in men. During pregnancy the level rises 2–3 fold and the rhythm disappears. Secretion is stimulated by TRH, phenothiazines, tricyclic drugs, methyl dopa and oestrogens and inhibited by L-dopa and bromocriptine.

Control of posterior pituitary function

ADH is controlled largely by osmoreceptors in the anterior hypothalamus, which operate in response to very small changes in osmolality of the plasma. Output of ADH is stimulated by a fall in plasma volume, by nicotine and some drugs; alcohol reduces ADH secretion.

The release of oxytocin is independent of ADH. The control system is at least partly neural as exemplified by the 'nipple' reflex whereby oxytocin is released rapidly when each act of suckling is begun.

Assessment of anterior pituitary function

This can be made at four different levels of complexity as appropriate for the circumstances, with more precise information appearing at successive levels.

Clinical

If a child is growing normally, with normal puberty, of if an adult is of normal height and weight with normal sexual function, any general pituitary defect is most unlikely.

Indirect

The secretion of most anterior pituitary hormones can be inferred from normal end organ function, viz:

T_4 plasma level	—TSH
Ovulation	—LH and FSH
Spermatogenesis	—LH and FSH
Cortisol plasma level	—ACTH
Bone age	—Related to sex hormones, T_4 and GH.

Direct, static

Routine assays are available for all the trophic hormones in plasma but isolated readings are of limited value because of wide fluctuations with time of day and circumstances.

TSH. Low levels are found in hyperthyroidism and raised levels in hypothyroidism.

LH and FSH. The normal levels are variable and relatively low compared with the sensitivity of current methods so that deficiency is not detected easily. FSH rises after the menopause and if the seminiferous tubules are badly damaged. LH rises sharply at the mid-peak of the menstrual cycle, after the menopause and with Leydig cell failure.

ACTH. This is unstable in transit so usually for convenience it is monitored indirectly by measurements of plasma cortisol which may indicate ACTH deficiency, excess and loss of diurnal rhythm.

GH. Normal fasting resting levels are higher in males (< 25 mu/l) than in females (< 15 mu/l).

PRL. Resting levels of PRL are a useful index in definite or suspected pituitary tumours and in the investigation of secondary amenorrhoea or infertility.

Direct, dynamic
There are many useful dynamic tests of trophic hormone release, but they are expensive and should only be used when clearly necessary.

TSH. Released after intravenous injection of TRH (see Chapter 6).

LH and FSH. Both released after intravenous injection of LHRH. Previous treatment with sex steroids may add further information.

ACTH. This is released after stress and various tests have been used. Insulin hypoglycaemia is favoured at present.

GH. Suppression of GH secretion occurs with a rise in blood glucose. This may be assessed during a standard glucose tolerance test (see Chapter 3 and below under 'Acromegaly'). Stimulation of GH release can be tested under many circumstances, e.g. sleep, oral hydrolysed protein, intravenous arginine and hypoglycaemia. The latter may be produced 4–5 h after a glucose load (a weak stimulus but entirely safe) or after insulin. A positive response to any stimulus is satisfactory evidence of normal GH secretion but a negative result is less definite. A failure to respond to at least two adequate stresses must be observed before it can be concluded that GH secretion is defective.

PRL. Release after TRH may be observed.

Testing in practice
The tests should be done in the morning with the patient rested and fasted. It is best to insert an indwelling venous cannula and take two

baseline specimens 15 min apart before applying the stimuli. *N.B.* If insulin is given, intravenous glucose and hydrocortisone must be immediately available and the patient must *never* be left unattended. After the test the patient *must* be fed and *not* released from supervision until all risk of hypoglycaemia has passed.

It is necessary to produce symptoms or signs of hypoglycaemia to ensure adequate stress but if the patient becomes distressed the hypoglycaemia can be terminated at once with i.v. glucose without reducing the usefulness of the results. The dose of insulin is 0.1 units to 0.3 units/ kg body weight—less in suspected hypopituitarism, more in obesity.

Combined testing
Because the trophic hormone systems are largely independent they can be tested individually but simultaneously. The stimuli can be given in sequence as slow intravenous injections of:

Soluble insulin (see above) from insulin syringe.
TRH 200 micrograms in 1 ml diluent.
LHRH 100 micrograms in 4 ml diluent.

Blood samples are taken after 20, 40 and 60 min for assays of LH, FSH, TSH, GH (PRL), glucose and cortisol. Alternatively, the tests can be done separately as necessary.

Interpretation of results
Basal levels will vary with circumstances. In general, at least a two-fold rise in hormone levels is to be expected in the normal but interpretation can be difficult. Usually these tests will not differentiate between hypothalamic and pituitary faults.

Assessment of posterior pituitary function

ADH
Plasma ADH can be measured by immunoassay. This is most usefully done during changes in water balance to observe whether ADH levels respond appropriately to changes in plasma osmolality.

Water deprivation test
The patient is weighed and bled, and then denied all moist food and fluid (under close supervision) for 8 hours. In the normal person after that time body weight will not have fallen by more than 3%, urine osmolality will be more than 600 mmol/kg and plasma osmolality

will not have risen above 300 mmol/kg. In ADH deficiency urine osmolality will be less than 300 mmol/kg and the plasma, more.

Diseases of the anterior pituitary gland

Although dysfunction of the hypothalmic-pituitary unit is common, particularly in respect of menstruation and fertility, major pituitary disease affecting general health is relatively rare.

HYPOPITUITARISM

When there is a general loss of anterior pituitary function, the term 'panhypopituitarism' is used. The loss of hormone secretion is by no means always uniform, thus varying the clinical features.

Clinical features

The presentation depends on the age of the patient. In children, slow growth in height and later a failure of puberty occur (see below). In middle age usually the onset is insidious with a failure of general health, loss of energy and slight weight gain with failure of menses or potency. In the older patient the features are even less definite and easily overlooked. Rarely, the patient presents more marked features of hypothyroidism or hypoadrenalism; coma may occur. On examination, the patient is lethargic with pallor due to a combination of anaemia and loss of pigmentation. Body, axillary and pubic hair is sparse or absent and in men the beard is sparse. The genitalia are atrophic but the breasts may appear normal. The speed of the tendon reflexes is slow (due to hypothyroidism) and the blood pressure tends to be low. Even if there is coincident damage to the neurohypophysis, diabetes insipidus does not occur because of cortisol deficiency.

Aetiology

Almost all the gland has to be destroyed before function is lost and at times the loss may be uneven.

Infarction. Severe obstetric shock and post-partum haemorrhage may cause infarction of the anterior pituitary (Sheehan's syndrome) which has enlarged during pregnancy. The condition may be apparent at once because of a failure of lactation and menses, or a pituitary remnant may remain which fails later. Infarction may follow meningitis, fracture of the skull or from cerebrovascular disease.

Destruction. The gland may be destroyed surgically, by implantation of radioactive seeds or external irradiation. Pressure from parapituitary tumours (e.g. craniopharyngioma) may cause hypopituitarism perhaps largely by damage to the hypothalamus. Pituitary tumours rarely cause hypopituitarism unless the tumour infarcts.

Finally, and rarely, the pituitary may be damaged by involvement with chronic granulomas, sarcoidosis or lipoidoses.

Diagnosis

This is suggested by evidence of end organ failure, e.g. reduced plasma levels of T_4 and cortisol with low plasma levels also of the trophic hormones. Blood glucose may be low and response to the various stimuli (see above) is lost. The changes may not be uniform and each function must be assessed separately. There may be evidence of generalised disease (e.g. sarcoid) and/or radiological evidence of bone destruction or calcification near the sella turcica.

Treatment

This consists of replacement therapy with the target organ hormones. It is important to start treatment with hydrocortisone and thyroxine together—if thyroxine is given alone, a hypoadrenal crisis may be provoked. Full doses of hydrocortisone, 30 mg per day and T_4 200 mg per day are suitable—there does not appear to be any need to begin treatment gradually. It is unlikely that any additional salt retaining steroid will be required but equally, the synthetic corticosteroids with little salt retaining power are usually unsuitable.

Treatment with sex steroids is indicated in the younger patient to restore libido. This therapy may have some protective action in the prevention of osteoporosis, but there is no evidence as to how long the treatment should be continued. Fertility may be possible with trophic hormones but for thyroid and adrenal replacement the trophic hormones are not used because of the inconvenience of injections.

Prognosis

This is essentially that of the underlying disease. The expectation of life in treated hypopituitarism is normal but extra steroid may be needed under stress.

Anorexia nervosa

The differential diagnosis of hypopituitarism and anorexia nervosa is sometimes mentioned, but should not present a problem, the only common feature being secondary amenorrhoea. In hypopituitarism, the appetite is poor but no worse, there is no aversion to food, no marked psychiatric features and rarely any weight loss. The behaviour of the patient with anorexia nervosa is the reverse of that in hypopituitarism, being alert and vivacious. Truncal hair is preserved and limb hair is increased. Subtle changes in hypothalamic-pituitary function have been detected in anorexia nervosa but it seems that they are secondary to starvation or the mental disease.

Selective hypopituitarism

Failure of secretion of one or more pituitary hormones may occur with preservation of the function of the rest of the gland. In some instances, the fault may be hypothalamic, particularly in respect of gonadotrophins. Isolated GH deficiency is also well known but the other isolated deficiencies are rare. The clinical features are those of failure of the target gland. The aetiology is unknown.

PITUITARY TUMOURS

These constitute about 10% of all intracranial tumours. As with tumours of other endocrine glands, the commonest form is the benign adenoma, but carcinomas may occur. Hormone secreting capacity is present in most adenomas and usually they escape from physiological control. The adenomas may be single or multiple and may or may not enlarge sufficiently to distend the sella turcica.

Pathology
The histological appearance of pituitary tumours is variable and often mixed. Tumours consisting mostly of chromophobe cells predominate but these may be secretory. Other tumours may consist predominantly of acidophil or basophil cells—the correlation between histology and function is not close. Hyaline change and fibrosis may occur, presumably the result of infarction.

Diagnosis
The presence of a tumour can be defined only by radiology or surgical exploration. Visual field defects without radiological change are unlikely. The biochemical function of the tumour may be assessed by the tests described above.

Radiology
A lateral 'coned' view of the sella turcica is suitable for screening or a

preliminary examination. The total area of the sella in the adult should not exceed 130 mm^2. The shape may be rounded suggesting distention even if the total area is normal. If the sella appears to have a 'double floor' this is evidence of asymmetrical expansion and the presence of a tumour. Usually, the posterior clinoids are preserved. Tomography may be able to delineate any upward extension of the tumour.

Local pressure

Most pituitary tumours are slow growing over many years. Prolonged pressure on the walls of the sella turcica leads to bone remodelling so that the fossa becomes dilated. The tumour may be asymmetrical in its downwards extension and also may spread upwards to involve the optic chiasma. Asymptomatic visual field defects may be detected by careful perimetry. The earliest loss is most likely to be in the superior temporal quadrants going on to full quadrantic defects and then bitemporal hemianopia. Raised intracranial pressure and papilloedema are rare.

Functional consequences of pituitary tumours

Various endocrine syndromes arise from pituitary tumours depending on which trophic hormone is secreted in excess. Usually, only one hormone is involved but very rarely there may be several. The remaining aspects of pituitary function are normal in many patients but sometimes, particularly with prolactin secreting tumours, other functions are affected. Panhypopituitarism may follow infarction.

Acromegaly—GH excess

This condition presents in either sex, usually in early or middle adult life, but very rarely the tumour arises in childhood causing gigantism. The presenting symptoms may be the change in facial appearance or the enlargement of hands and feet. A carpal tunnel syndrome is common and the patient may report excessive sweating, loss of libido or changes in the menses. Other features may include arthritis, backache or visual field defects. On examination the appearance is characteristic in most patients. Inspection of old photographs may help. The tissues of the face are coarse, thickened or folded so that deep clefts appear. The nose, lips and tongue are thickened. Enlargement of the jaw gives a forward bite and the hands are large with broad fingers. The thoracic cage may be large and the liver palpable. Radiographs show enlargement of the jaw and frontal sinuses, and 'tufting' of the terminal phalanges. The heel pad is thickened and usually the sella turcica is enlarged.

Biochemical tests

The diagnosis is established by showing an elevated level of plasma growth hormone which is not suppressed (or may even rise) after glucose loading (Fig. 8.5). The incidence of clinical diabetes mellitus is somewhat increased. A glucose tolerance test shows minor loss of tolerance in about half of the patients.

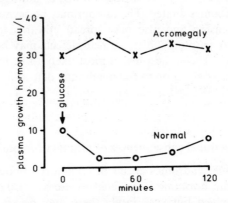

FIG. 8.5. Typical response of plasma growth hormone during a standard 50 g oral glucose tolerance test. Some acromegalics have much higher levels but all have lost the suppressibility of growth hormone which is seen in the normal.

Treatment

The best treatment for acromegaly is disputed—all the techniques described below have been used alone or in combination. Recently, bromocriptine has been tried with occasional success but evaluation is still incomplete. When GH levels are lowered there is a shrinkage of soft tissues, relief of symptoms and improvement in carbohydrate tolerance but clinical diabetes is not necessarily relieved. Reversal of bone changes is very slow.

Long-term follow-up is essential. GH levels should be measured regularly because the results of treatment are uncertain. Sometimes GH declines over months or years, particularly after radiotherapy, but sometimes it rises and further treatment is needed. Also, the function of the rest of the anterior pituitary may change so review of replacement therapy is important.

Prognosis

No specific acromegalic heart disease can be established but it is known that life expectancy is reduced in untreated acromegaly and that the increased mortality is due to cardiovascular causes. If GH levels are high, treatment is recommended to prolong life and prevent deformity.

Cushing's disease

This is due to excess secretion of ACTH. Many of the patients have basophilic microadenomas and a few have large tumours. Hypophysectomy is a possible form of treatment (see Chapter 9).

Prolactinomas

Many pituitary tumours previously thought to be functionless in fact secrete PRL. Microadenomas may be responsible also. Presentation is with infertility, amenorrhoea and/or galactorrhoea (see Chapter 13).

Miscellaneous

Pituitary tumours may very rarely secrete other hormones including TSH causing hyperthyroidism. A tumour secreting ADH has not been described.

HYPOPHYSECTOMY

The application of procedures to destroy all or part of the pituitary gland is now quite common, although the best method in various circumstances is disputed. In the case of tumours the ideal treatment would destroy the tumour and leave the remaining gland intact but this is difficult to achieve. Complete ablation is sought to try to ensure complete destruction of a tumour. Four main treatments have been used.

Surgical; transcranial
The operation is a craniotomy with removal of the tumour from above. This method is essential if the tumour extends much above the sella to involve the chiasma but otherwise alternative methods are preferred.

Surgical; trans-sphenoidal
This technique involves approaching the sella turcica through the sphenoid sinus and the removal of the front wall of the sella. Meticulous

anaesthetic technique with hypotension is essential. Microdissection of the gland for removal of microadenomas has been reported.

External irradiation

This may be carried out with ortho- or megavoltage therapy, or proton beam. There is some risk of damage to the brain. Irradiation may be applied after surgery. When used alone the results are mixed, largely because of the difficulty of delivering safely an adequate dose to such a deep structure. Hormone secretion from tumours does fall but this may be slow and take several years.

Internal irradiation

This involves the implantation of radioactive seeds (e.g. ^{90}Yttrium) into the gland via a needle through the sphenoid sinus.

Post-operative hormone replacement

For the surgical procedures, hydrocortisone is given before the operation and continued afterwards. In about half the patients there is a transient diabetes insipidus requiring treatment with ADH but this condition remits after a few weeks. What other hormone replacement is needed later can be determined only by trial in the individual patient. After all these treatments, whether by design or accident, there may be considerable residual pituitary function and even normal menses and pregnancy. Careful follow-up examinations with hormone measurements and observations of the effects of gradual withdrawal of replacement therapy will define the situation. If in doubt, replacement with hydrocortisone and thyroxine (as in panhypopituitarism) should be given. Even if no regular replacement is needed, stress response may be inadequate. Sex hormone replacement may be needed.

DIABETES INSIPIDUS

This is the only recognised form of posterior pituitary deficiency and is due to ADH lack. The clinical features are polyuria, with a urine flow of 5 to 10 litres per day and consequent dehydration thirst and sleep disturbance. There are no specific physical signs but features related to an underlying disease may be found.

Pathology

In many patients there is no obvious cause but in others there is evident damage to the pituitary and/or hypothalmus. Causes include primary and secondary tumours in or near the pituitary fossa, trauma, sarcoidosis, meningitis, and the lipoidoses. Destruction of the posterior pituitary alone causes only transient diabetes insipidus. If anterior pituitary adrenocorticotrophic function is lost as well as ADH secretion, diabetes insipidus does not appear because of the effect of cortisol deficiency on renal function. The administration of corticosteroids will unmask the diabetes insipidus. Adequate levels of cortisol must be assured before tests for diabetes insipidus can be carried out reliably.

Diagnosis

The differential diagnosis includes diabetes mellitus, nephrogenic diabetes insipidus (in which the nephron is resistant to the action of ADH and which may be due to the administration of lithium), chronic renal disease and compulsive water drinking. The latter is a psychological disorder which may give difficulties in diagnosis but the appropriate test should show normal ADH response. Also, the administration of ADH to these patients is followed by a continued high fluid intake and water intoxication whereas in diabetes insipidus the improvement with ADH is immediate and dramatic. The water deprivation test should establish the diagnosis but alternatively ADH assay compared with changes in osmolality may be used.

Treatment

The best preparation is a long acting synthetic analogue of vasopressin called *desmopressin* which is taken usually as a nasal spray in a dose of 10–20 mg once or twice a day. It may be injected intravenously or intramuscularly in a dose of 1–2 mg also once or twice a day.

Aqueous vasopressin is available for subcutaneous or intramuscular injection. The dose is 5–10 units and the effect lasts only a few hours. The analogue lysine vasopressin can be taken as a nasal spray in a dose of 10–20 units every few hours.

There are non-hormonal drugs which may achieve quite good control of urine output in diabetes insipidus. Paradoxically, diuretics may be used but chlorpropamide is better although it carries some risk of hypoglycaemia. Carbamazepine has been used also.

SYNDROME OF INAPPROPRIATE ADH SECRETION '(SIADH)'

This strange condition presents clinically with the features of water intoxication, i.e. anorexia, nausea, vomiting, headache, weakness and confusion going on to coma. Oedema is unusual. The aetiology is obscure. There is an excess of ADH but its origin is uncertain. SIADH may occur in association with carcinoma of the bronchus and other non-pituitary tumours which are synthesising ADH or a similar substance. The syndrome can occur also with non-malignant conditions of the lung, e.g. pneumonia and tuberculosis, as well as many general or CNS diseases including encephalitis, head injury, cerebrovascular accidents and brain tumours. In these instances the ADH is released presumably from the neurohypophysis.

Diagnosis
This is established indirectly. The plasma osmolality is low (less than 270 mmol/kg) and the urine osmolality is greater than that of the plasma; ADH assay should be helpful. Also, the urine sodium is high despite a low level in the plasma; this is unexplained.

Treatment
Water restriction to an intake of 500 to 1000 ml per day is effective; some degree of water restriction may be needed long-term. The drug demeclocycline has been used with benefit. The underlying disease is treated and if a tumour can be removed or successfully irradiated the SIADH remits.

SHORT STATURE

There is no precise definition of short stature. If the possibility is raised the patient's height must be compared with standard charts for age and sex, including allowance for the height of the parents if that is out of the ordinary. The charts* prepared by Tanner *et al.* are excellent. If the height is below the third percentile (i.e. about 2 S.D's below the mean) the situation merits investigation. It is most important that unusually short children are identified early, i.e. below 7 years of age, to allow proper advice and treatment where possible. Clinical examination may reveal underlying disease, e.g. cyanotic congenital heart disease, pale optic discs, skeletal disproportion and deformity or mental retardation. In older children puberty may be delayed.

Aetiology
The classification of causes of short stature is unsatisfactory and somewhat arbitrary.

* Available from Creaseys of Hertford Ltd, Castlemead, Hertford, U.K.

Genetic. 'Constitutional' (the commonest cause)
  Familial (inherited from short stature parents)
  Achondroplasia
  Turner's syndrome

Nutritional or general. Low birth weight and subsequent slow growth (? intra-uterine malnutrition).
  General severe disease e.g. congenital heart disease, renal disease, cystic fibrosis, chronic infection, collagenosis, mental retardation, coeliac disease, rickets, diabetes.

Social. Severe emotional deprivation which supresses growth hormone release.

Endocrine. Isolated GH deficiency
  Panhypopituitarism (due usually to craniopharyngioma)
  Hypothyroidism
  Hypercortisolism
  Precocious puberty

Diagnosis
The following scheme of investigation should establish the diagnosis in the large majority of patients.

History. Particular attention to parents height, birth weight, growth history, social circumstances, behaviour and school record.

Physical examination. Body proportions: short limbs may indicate achondroplasia. Skeletal deformities such as short metatarsals, increased carrying angle and webbed neck suggest Turner's syndrome. Cyanosis and signs of heart disease may be present. Hypothyroidism may be evident.

Investigations. 1. Radiographs of hand and wrist for skeletal maturity (see reference) and of sella turcica. If skeletal maturity (bone age) is consistent with chronological age, growth hormone deficiency is unlikely. Chest X-ray for chronic lung disease.
2. Haematology. Low haemoglobin and plasma iron may indicate coeliac disease. Polycythaemia may indicate cyanotic heart disease.
3. Biochemistry. Blood urea, electrolytes and calcium to seek chronic renal or coeliac disease.
4. Genetic investigations. A buccal smear examination for sex chroma-

tin is essential in all female patients and should be supported by chromosome analysis.

5. Endocrine investigation. Serum T_4 and TSH for hypothyroidism. Plasma cortisol also if panhypopituitarism is suspected.

6. Growth hormone. Fasting resting plasma GH measurements are often low in normal children so single readings in these circumstances are unhelpful. It is necessary to demonstrate whether there is GH response to above 20 mu/l to exclude GH deficiency—various test situations have been devised (see above in assessment of pituitary function). A poor GH response may be due to a generalised disease.

7. Miscellaneous. Initial clues may indicate further tests, e.g. small intestinal biopsy for coeliac disease or a sweat test for cystic fibrosis. Other tests of pituitary function may be indicated.

Treatment
This follows from the diagnosis but many patients cannot be treated successfully, particularly if diagnosed late. Children with GH deficiency may be considered for treatment by human GH injections. In older children the administration of sex hormones may be requested but this is undesirable as they produce a growth spurt followed by epiphyseal fusion so that adult height may be reduced even further.

EXCESSIVE HEIGHT

This is an uncommon complaint but occasionally children are presented for treatment who are growing very quickly and appear likely to reach an excessive adult height. Often the parents are tall. In these circumstances it is desirable to exclude the very rare pituitary tumour with growth hormone excess but almost always the cause will be constitutional. Treatment is not essential but is requested for cosmetic reasons. The expected adult height may be estimated from tables using the patient's bone age, and height, and parents height (see references and footnote on p. 126). With discussion, the parents may agree that no treatment is required. If necessary, premature puberty may be induced in boys with androgens and girls with a combination of oestrogen and progestogen. These treatments cause premature closure of the epiphyses and early cessation of growth. There is no evidence that these treatments are harmful but such early hormonal manipulation seems undesirable on general principles.

REFERENCES

TANNER J.M. *et al.* (1975). *Assessment of Skeletal Maturity and Prediction of Adult Height (TW2 Method).* Academic Press, London.
VIGNERI R. & GOLDFINE I.D. (1980). Pharmacologic therapy of patients with pituitary tumors secreting prolactin, growth hormone and adrenocorticotrophin. *Advances in Internal Medicine*, **25**, 69.
ZERBE R. *et al.* (1980). Vasopressin function in the syndrome of inappropriate antidiuresis. *Annual Review of Medicine*, **31**, 315.

FURTHER READING

ABBOUD C.F. & LAWS E.R. (1979). Clinical endocrinological approach to hypothalamic-pituitary disease. *Journal of Neurosurgery*, **51**, 271.
DONALD R.A. (1980). ACTH and related peptides. *Clinical Endocrinology*, **12**, 491.
FRANKS S. *et al* (1977) Prevalence and presentation of hyperprolactinaemia in patients with 'functionless' pituitary tumours. *Lancet, i*, 778.
FRASIER S.D. (1979). Growth disorders in children. *Paediatric Clinics of North America*, **26**, (*1*) 3.
HANKINSON J. & BANNA M. (1976). *Pituitary and Parapituitary Tumours.* Saunders, London.
MILNER R.D.G. *et al* (1979). Experience with human growth hormone in Great Britain. *Clinical Endocrinology*, **11**, 15.
SCHALLY A. V. *et al* (1978). Hypothalamic regulatory hormones. *Annual Review of Biochemistry*, **47**, 89.
TANNER J.M. *et al* (1966). Standards from birth to maturity for height, weight, height velocity and weight velocity. *Archives Diseases of Childhood*, **41**, 454, 613.

Chapter 9
Adrenal

ANATOMY

The adrenal glands each weigh about 5 g in the adult and they lie over the upper poles of the kidneys. The *medulla* or inner part produces catecholamines and the *cortex* or outer part produces steroids. Although their proximity and some structural features suggest a functional link the two parts act largely independently and cause distinctive diseases.

ADRENAL CORTEX

Physiology

Chemistry

The cells of the adrenal cortex can synthesise cholesterol and also take it up from the circulation. Cholesterol is converted to Δ^{5-} pregnenolone from which all the corticosteroids are derived. The nomenclature of the steroids is complex and only some of the simpler rules and 'trivial' names are given here. The numbering of the parent molecule is shown in Fig. 9.1. The number in the names of steroids may refer to the total number of carbon atoms (e.g. C_{21}—seventeen in the rings plus four in the side chains) or a position in the molecule (e.g. OH-11—a hydroxyl group at the eleven position). Stereoisomerism in the 'trans' or 'cis' configuration occurs between 'A' and 'B' rings. Side chains are designated 'β' (and indicated conventionally in diagrams by a solid line) if they project on the same side of the plane of the ring as the 19-methyl group. Side chains projecting on the opposite side are called 'α' (and indicated by a dotted line). A double bond in a ring is referred to as '-ene' and by the number of the carbon at which it originates. It is understood to terminate at the next higher numbered carbon atom. Thus, '5-ene' means a double bond between C-5 and C-6; it may also be written 'Δ^5'. 'Oxo' means an oxygen atom attached by a double bond at the position indicated. Oxosteroids used to be called ketosteroids.

Many steroids have been isolated from the adrenal cortex but only three are of major importance.

Cortisol (hydrocortisone). About 70 μmol are secreted each day, mostly from the zona fasciculata (central layer) and the zona reticularis (inner layer). Cortisol is C_{21}, OH-11.

Dehydroepiandrosterone (DHA). This is secreted from the same layers and in about the same amount as cortisol. It is C_{19}, O-17.

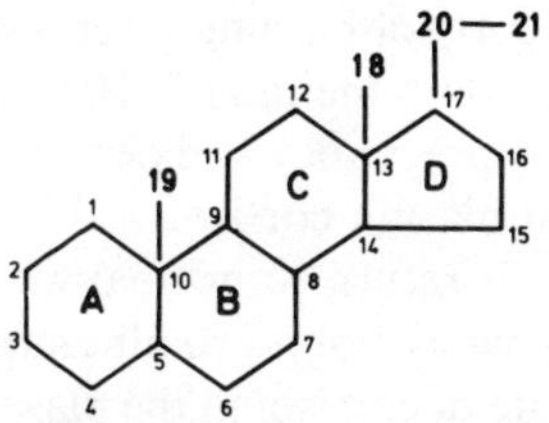

FIG. 9.1 The cyclopentanophenanthrene ring and some side chains. The letters refer to the rings and the numbers to carbon atoms.

Aldosterone. About 400 nmol are secreted each day, mostly from the zona glomerulosa (outer layer). It is a C_{21}, CHO-18. Some corticosterone is produced and also a little testosterone and oestrogens.

The release of cortisol into the circulation is intermittent resulting in sudden large rises in plasma level with subsequent decay. Possibly other corticosteroids are released similarly.

Control of corticosteroid secretion
The structure of the adrenal cortex is maintained by ACTH which also stimulates the synthesis and release of cortisol, DHA and some other corticosteroids. The zona glomerulosa and aldosterone secretion are largely independent of ACTH action. The secretion of cortisol is controlled by three systems acting simultaneously.
1. Superimposed on the pulsatile release there is a diurnal rhythm of secretion producing a maximum plasma level at about 0600 h with a fall to about half the maximum by 2200 h. The rhythm is intrinsic in the brain but triggered by light; it is mediated through the hypothalamus, CRH and ACTH.
2. There is a response to mental or physical stress, also via CRH and ACTH. The response time is a few minutes only and there is sufficient stored cortisol to raise the plasma level by twofold or more. Synthesis can increase quickly also.
3. There is a feedback loop with modulation of ACTH secretion by cortisol (and synthetic glucocorticoids) but other steroid products of the cortex do not have this effect.
   Aldosterone secretion is controlled largely by angiotensin II from the renin-angiotensin system (see below). It is stimulated in many situations including upright posture, haemorrhage, dehydration, sodium loss or restriction of intake and potassium loading.

Corticosteroid metabolism
After release, about 75% of cortisol is bound in the circulation to transcortin, a specific cortisol binding glycoprotein. A further 15% is bound to albumin and the remaining 5–10% is free. Plasma levels of transcortin are raised by pregnancy and oestrogen administration causing an increase in total plasma cortisol with little evidence of cortisol excess. Transcortin levels return to normal when oestrogens are withdrawn. Aldosterone is partly bound to albumin; the carriage of DHA is uncertain. The half-life of cortisol in the plasma is about 90 min. It is degraded, mainly in the liver, by enzymatic reduction of the Δ^4 bond and also modification of the O-3 group to OH-3.

Other corticosteroids are metabolised similarly but alternative metabolic pathways have been identified. The degraded products are biologically inert. They are conjugated with glucuronic, phosphoric or sulphuric acid and excreted in the urine. Aldosterone is metabolised similarly to cortisol but DHA is partly sulphonated and this compound tends to remain in the circulation bound to protein. Apart from the traces of free corticosteroids which enter the urine, they are excreted by the kidney in conjugated form; the steroid nucleus cannot be degraded.

Actions of steroids
Many effects of corticosteroids have been found and minor alterations in the molecules can produce profound changes in their actions; they may have varying potencies in different respects. This has been exploited by the production of synthetic steroids which retain some properties but not others, to increase their value in therapy. Some actions however, cannot be separated. It is important to distinguish the physiological actions of corticosteroids from the pharmacological ones, which appear when larger amounts are present.

Glucocorticoid effect. The major action is to promote gluconeogenesis and antagonise insulin action to maintain plasma glucose levels. Liver glycogen is maintained also. Water diuresis, white cell numbers and blood pressure are supported. The physiological role of the diurnal fluctuations of plasma cortisol (the natural adrenal glucocorticoid) is uncertain but it might have had survival value in primitive man. Excess glucocorticoid effect leads to:

Hyperglycaemia, nitrogen wasting, increased fat synthesis and hyperlipaemia.
Inhibition of growth, osteoporosis, tissue fragility.
Inhibition of the inflammatory response and subsequent fibrosis.
Suppression of ACTH release.
Suppression of vitamin D action.
Changes in mood with elation and occasionally psychosis; muscle weakness.

Mineralo-corticoid effect. This is a direct action on ion transport by epithelial cells, particularly in the distal renal tubule, resulting in sodium conservation and potassium excretion. Excess effect is an exaggeration of these changes leading to oedema and hypertension. Aldosterone produces 75% of the mineralo-corticoid effect in man. The other 25% is caused by cortisol, which is a relatively weak mineralo-corticoid but is present in much larger amounts.

Sex hormone effects. The traces of oestrogen produced by the adrenal cortex are of little importance. DHA although a weak androgen is produced in large amounts. It is of no significance in the normal male because its effect is swamped by that of testosterone but at puberty DHA may aid the development of sexual hair and in the post menopausal women it may help to maintain the skeleton. These effects are slight and DHA is not necessary for normal health. It is mysterious why a material of such little apparent use should be produced in such large quantities.

Synthetic corticosteroids

Manipulation of the steroid molecule has produced chemicals with widely varying ratios of glucocorticoid/mineralo-corticoid effect (see Table 9.1). At the extremes, in comparison with cortisol, fludrocortisone has a ratio of 0·025 and dexamethasone a ratio of 15.

So far no compound has been produced in which the valuable anti-inflammatory action has been separated from other glucocorticoid effects and all the synthetic corticosteroids have the same potentially dangerous side effect.

TABLE. 9.1. Approximate relative potencies on a weight basis of some natural and synthetic corticosteroids.

Steroid	Glucocorticoid (anti-inflammatory) effect	Mineralocorticoid (salt retaining) effect
Cortisone/cortisol	1	1
Prednisone/prednisolone	5	1
Dexamethasone	30	2
Fludrocortisone	10	400

Cortisone. This compound is O-11 whereas cortisol is OH-11 but otherwise they are identical. Cortisone is converted rapidly to cortisol by a liver enzyme so the administration of cortisone produces cortisol in the plasma.

Glucocorticoids. The most widely used are prednisone and prednisolone which are identical to cortisone and cortisol respectively except that both contain a Δ^1. It is likely that prednisone is converted to prednisolone in the liver; therapeutically they are identical. Other more potent glucocorticoids have no advantage in general use except in tests.

Topical and local corticosteroids. Other synthetic corticosteroids and/or their derivatives are valuable for special uses such as intra-articular injection or topical application.

Mineralo-corticoid. Cortisol with a fluorine atom at '9α' makes 9α-fluorocortisol which has been given the confusing pharmacopoeial name of 'fludrocortisone'. It is used as a substitute for aldosterone.

Renin-angiotensin system

Renin is an enzyme released from the juxta-glomerular apparatus which comprises some structures at the vascular pole of the glomerulus. In the plasma, renin acts on a substrate (angiotensinogen) which is an α_2 globulin, to release the relatively inert decapeptide, angiotensin I. A 'converting enzyme' in the plasma removes two terminal amino acids leaving the octapeptide angiotensin II. This is supposed to be the active substance although further conversion has been postulated. Angiotensin II has a pressor effect by direct action on the vascular bed but acts also on the zona glomerulosa to promote the synthesis and release of aldosterone (Fig. 9.2). This is probably the main determinant of aldosterone secretion. The release of renin is stimulated by many situations but particularly upright posture, haemorrhage, dehydration, sodium loss or restriction, potassium loading, renal ischaemia, hepatic cirrhosis, congestive cardiac failure and hypoalbuminaemia. The secretion of renin is suppressed by angiotensin II but it seems likely that other parts of the feedback system remain to be discovered.

The relevance of the renin-angiotensin system to clinical practice at present, even in connection with hypertension, is small.

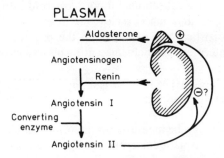

FIG. 9.2. The renal-adrenal cycle of the renin-angiotensin-aldosterone system. The control 'loop' may be completed by angiotensin II suppressing the release of renin.

Tests of adrenocortical function

Many different methods of estimation of corticosteroids have been developed. Most of them measure groups of compounds but specific methods for individual compounds are preferred.

Plasma

Cortisol is best measured by immunoassay. Because of the episodic release of cortisol the plasma level may vary considerably and surprisingly low readings may be recorded in normal people. Repeated measurements may be essential and also specimens in the morning and evening to plot the diurnal variation. Emotional stress raises plasma cortisol so out-patient readings may be falsely high.

Aldosterone can be measured by immunoassay also. The patient must be prepared with care to ensure basal results. Diuretics and some other drugs must be discontinued for at least three weeks previously. A diet containing at least 100 mmol of sodium and 50 mmol of potassium per day must be taken for three days. The specimen is taken in the early morning after an overnight rest and before the patient moves from the horizontal position.

17-α-Hydroxyprogesterone. This assay is now available and may prove useful for the investigation of adrenal enzyme deficiencies (below).

ACTH. This assay is particularly useful in the differential diagnosis of Cushing's syndrome.

Urine
The use of 24 h urine collections for corticosteroid assays entails obvious disadvantages and inaccuracies but does provide measures of average adrenocortical activity through the day and overcomes the difficulties of interpreting widely fluctuating plasma levels.

Cortisol. Small amounts of free cortisol appear in the urine and can be measured readily.

Aldosterone. This can be measured in the urine but all the precautions given above for plasma aldosterone (except recumbency) must be observed.

Oxygenation index. This is the ratio of two fractions of the urinary 17-oxogenic steroids. The '11-deoxy' fraction is derived from cortisol precursors, mostly pregnanetriol, while OH-11 fraction is from cortisol. The 11-oxygenation index is '11-deoxy/OH-11. Various methods of estimating the fractions have been used. Any fresh specimen of urine is acceptable without a timed collection. The test is helpful in detecting adrenal enzyme faults (see adrenogenital syndrome).

The measurement of total 17-oxosteroids and 17-oxogenic steroids in the urine is being replaced by more reliable plasma assays.

Dynamic tests
As with many endocrine tests, additional important imformation can be gained by measuring hormone levels in varying circumstances.

Stimulation tests

Using ACTH. This test examines the responsiveness of the adrenal cortex to ACTH. A convenient short test is as follows; it is best done in the morning. Blood is taken before and thirty minutes after an intramuscular injection of 250 mg of aqueous tetracosactrin. In the normal person the plasma cortisol should show an increment of at least 200 nmol/l and reach a level of at least 600 nmol/l. More prolonged stimulation with depot injections may be employed.

Using stress. This tests capacity of the pituitary to release ACTH and the response of the adrenal cortex. Of the various stresses hypoglycaemia after insulin is favoured at present (see Chapter 8).

Using metabolic blockade. Metyrapone inhibits the $11-\beta$ hydroxylase of the adrenal cortex. When the drug is given, cortisol synthesis is impeded, plasma cortisol falls, ACTH release is stimulated and corticosteroid synthesis is increased. The increased steroids have to bypass the cortisol pathway but appear in the urine. A normal response to metyrapone is an increase in urinary 17-oxogenic steroids.

Suppression tests
These are used to determine the extent to which corticosteroid production remains under physiological control. It is usual to administer dexamethasone because its high potency permits a low dose by weight and therefore less risk of interference in the measurement of the endogenous steroids. In the normal, the dexamethasone suppresses ACTH release and adrenocortical secretion is reduced. Two tests are in general use.

Short test. Plasma cortisol is measured at about 0900 h on two successive mornings. At the midnight between the two samples, dexamethasone 1 mg is given by mouth. If the patient is more than 20% above their ideal body weight, the dose should be 2 mg. In the normal person the second plasma cortisol is reduced by at least half to below 300 nmol/l.

Long test (Liddle test). Plasma cortisol is measured at 0900 h each day; urine free cortisol may be used instead. The schedule is as follows:

Day 1 control
Day 2 control
Day 3 dexamethasone 0.5 mg, 6 hourly by mouth
Day 4 dexamethasone 0.5 mg, 6 hourly by mouth
Day 5 dexamethasone 2.0 mg, 6 hourly by mouth
Day 6 dexamethasone 2.0 mg, 6 hourly by mouth.

In the normal plasma cortisol falls to low levels on both doses of dexamethasone. In patients with Cushing's syndrome due to excessive production of ACTH by the pituitary, the lower dose of dexamethasone has no effect but the higher dose does suppress ACTH release and reduces the cortisol. Excess corticosteroid production due to the ectopic ACTH syndrome or an adrenal tumour is not affected by either dose of dexamethasone.

The reliability of the adrenocortical function tests are discussed in connection with their appliction. Approximate normal values are given in table 9.2.

TABLE. 9.2. Approximate normal values for various corticosteroids

Specimen	Corticosteroid	Normal values	Units
Plasma/Serum	Cortisol	0900 h 300–700	nmol/l
		2200 h < 200	nmol/l
Plasma/Serum	Aldosterone*	< 800	pmol/l
Plasma/Serum	ACTH	0900 h 10–80	ng/l
		2200 h < 10	ng/l
Urine	Free cortisol	100–500	nmol/24 h
Urine	Aldosterone (total)	10–30	nmol/24 h
Urine	11 deoxy.	1.5–10.0 (adults)	nmol/24 h
Urine	OH-11	7–24 (adults)	nmol/24 h
Urine	oxygenation index	< 0.7 (adults)	—

* See Text for precautions.

DISEASES OF THE ADRENAL CORTEX

Cushing's syndrome

This condition is due to excessive secretion of adrenocortical steroids, particularly cortisol. Most of the clinical features can be produced by the administration of pharmacological doses of synthetic corticosteroids. The disease is rare, occurring usually in early or middle adult life and much more commonly in women than men.

Clinical

The onset is slow over months or years and the condition may fluctuate. The symptoms are variable but include weight gain, secondary amenorrhoea and infertility, muscular weakness, change in facial appearance, and the symptoms of hypertension and diabetes. In addition there may be backache, bruising, striae, acne and hirsutism. Mental changes, ranging from lability of mood to psychosis are common.

The appearance of a patient with florid Cushing's syndrome is striking. Usually there is moderate or severe obesity and the face is round and red ('moon face'). The musculature is poor and the subcutaneous fat has an abnormal distribution being relatively thicker than normal over the trunk and thinner over the limbs. Pads of fat may be obvious over the upper dorsal spine and above the clavicles. The skin is thin with easy bruising and pink striae caused by tearing of the subcutaneous tissues. The striae tend to lie across the lines of skin tension, appearing on the sides of the abdomen, breasts, thighs, buttocks, hips and axillary folds. Acne and some excess body and facial hair may be present. There may be slight enlargment of the clitoris. The blood pressure is raised and complications of hypertension may be present. Radiographs may show osteoporosis and, in a few patients, enlargement of the sella turcica.

Sometimes the clinical features are not so obvious. The fat distribution may be normal and body weight only slightly increased. The diagnosis should be considered in patients presenting with hypertension and diabetes, obesity particularly with striae, hirsutism and/or virilism and obesity with psychosis.

Pathology

There are no specific histological changes except in the pituitary and adrenal. Non-specific changes include hypertensive cardiomegaly and osteoporosis. A glucose tolerance test may show a diabetic curve.

Aetiology

Four types are recognised.

Cushing's disease. This accounts for about 80% of the patients. It may be that the primary fault is hypothalamic but this is unproven. Certainly the anterior pituitary is involved and secretes an excess of ACTH. Histologically the pituitary may show focal concentrations of basiphils or a small basiphilic adenoma. The basiphil cells show degranulation (Crooke's change) but this is secondary to glucocorticoid excess. Rarely, there is a tumour large enough to distend the fossa. There is bilateral hyperplasia of the adrenal cortex.

Adrenal tumour. This is present in about 15% of patients. Usually it is a single benign adenoma but corticosteroid secreting carcinomas occur. The metastases may secrete also. Bilateral tumours may occur.

Ectopic ACTH. One of the best known syndromes of ectopic hormone production is that of ACTH release from malignant tumours of non-endocrine origin usually an oat-celled bronchial carcinoma. Most such patients do not show the typical features of Cushing's syndrome and the clinical picture is characterised by the rapid progression of a severe illness, weight loss, oedema, pigmentation and hypokalaemia.

Alcoholism. This can cause a transient syndrome indistinguishable from Cushing's disease.

Diagnosis
The initial diagnosis of Cushing's syndrome depends on the demonstration of excessive secretion of cortisol. The interpretation of the tests described above is less straightforward than is sometimes claimed. The normal ranges are wide and vary with circumstances.

The plasma cortisol is the best screening test but slightly raised levels occur in obesity and if the patient is stressed. The morning levels of plasma cortisol may be almost normal in Cushing's syndrome but the diurnal rhythm is lost and the demonstration of this lack is useful but not diagnostic. Such a lack may be caused by a low calorie diet in an obese patient. A failure of suppression with a midnight dose of dexamethasone is helpful also. Urine 17-steroid estimations are unreliable unless very high; they are increased somewhat in simple obesity. Urine free cortisol is better and gives an approximate indication of cortisol production rate. Repeated observations of steroid levels may be needed. The presence of osteoporosis and impaired glucose tolerance may help.

Aetiological diagnosis
Once cortisol excess has been demonstrated, an aetiological diagnosis is required to direct treatment. The level of plasma ACTH is low in adrenal tumour, raised in Cushing's disease and very high in the ectopic ACTH syndrome—probably this is the best single test. The presence of a hypokalaemic alkalosis suggests ectopic ACTH production.

The long dexamethasone suppression test is fairly reliable at differentiating adrenal tumour from Cushing's disease and metyrapone may be useful also but all the tests fail on occasions. The finding of a carcinoma, e.g. in the lung, may settle the question. Direct investigation of the adrenals is discussed below.

Treatment

An adrenal tumour should be removed but the other adrenal will be atrophic. Corticosteroid replacement will be needed for months and withdrawn gradually to restore normal adrenal function. An obvious pituitary tumour should be dealt with by external radiation, implantation or trans-sphenoidal hypophysectomy. The treatment of Cushing's disease without an obvious pituitary tumour is more controversial; sub-total adrenalectomy is likely to be of only temporary benefit. Total adrenalectomy is the usual treatment and cure is virtually guaranteed but the operation is hazardous and post-operative shock, sepsis and delayed healing may be troublesome. Permanent corticosteroid replacement is needed. A late complication is Nelson's syndrome; this condition is caused by an enlarging pituitary tumour, usually with intense skin pigmentation, years after total adrenalectomy. It is presumed that there is continued growth of a pituitary adenoma which was causing the Cushing's disease.

An alternative treatment of Cushing's disease is pituitary destruction by various means (See Chapter 8). Cure is less certain but the treatment is safer and the risk of Nelson's syndrome is removed.

Medical treatment

There are three drugs currently available which will suppress cortisol secretion, namely, metyrapone, aminoglutethimide and trilostane. They may be used to control Cushing's syndrome (and therefore reduce operative risk) before radical therapy or as an alternative if such treatment is not possible.

Prognosis

Untreated Cushing's syndrome is fatal in a few years from cardiovascular disease or sepsis. After radical treatment the outlook is good, depending on whether there has been irreversible cardiovascular damage.

Permanent replacement treatment carries some risk at times of stress and special care is needed. Adrenal or other carcinomas are likely to be rapidly fatal from cachexia and/or metastases.

Andrenogenital syndromes

These uncommon disorders are due to a complete or partial lack of one or more of the specific enzymes required for steroid synthesis. The cause is genetic and the usual inheritance is autosomal recessive. The main effect of the fault is on the adrenal but sometimes the gonads are affected also. Many types have been described; only the best known are described here. Figure 9.3. shows the enzymes concerned.

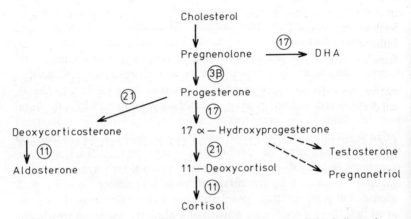

Fig. 9.3. An outline of steroid synthesis. The numbers in circles indicate the enzymes involved. The pathways marked with interrupted lines are quantitatively small in the normal but increase when the C–21 or C–11 enzymes are deficient.

Clinical features

These vary widely depending on the location and severity of the enzyme fault. In general, the changes are due to combinations of cortisol and aldosterone lack, mineralo-corticoid excess and androgen excess. The cortisol deficiency stimulates ACTH release which leads to adrenal hyperplasia—hence the alternative name 'congenital adrenal hyperplasia'—and excess steroid production. Because of the enzyme deficiency the steroids are deflected into pathways which are normally minor, and an abnormal pattern of steroid production results. All the patients have normal male or female genotype and usually normal differentiation of the gonads and internal sexual organs but the other sexual characteristics are variable. The condition presents in four major forms:

1. In the female neonate with ambiguous external genitalia ('female pseudo-hermaphroditism').
2. Severe disease in neonates of both sexes with a salt losing state or hypertension.

3. Precocious virilisation with small testicles in young boys and virilisation in young girls.
4. Primary amenorrhoea with virilisation in older girls.

Pathology
The major defects which have been defined are:

C-20 hydroxylase deficiency. This is the most severe type. The defect is in a very early stage of steroid synthesis. The gonads are affected as well so that sex hormone synthesis is defective. Consequently, male infants lack intrauterine testosterone and their external genitalia are female in form so all these patients appear female at birth.

The adrenal glands are engorged with cholesterol; hence the alternative name 'lipoid adrenal hyperplasia'. With such a severe biochemical defect it is not surprising that usually the condition is quickly lethal.

C-3β dehydrogenase deficiency. This defect also affects the gonads; there is a deficiency of cortisol, aldosterone and testosterone but an excess of DHA so that the external genitalia are ambiguous in both sexes.

C-17α hydroxylase deficiency. This defect also affects the gonads. Cortisol is deficient but corticosterone secretion is increased so that salt retention and hypertension occurs. Females have normal external genitalia but do not menstruate—males have pseudo-hermaphroditism.

C-21 hydroxylase deficiency. This is the commonest type. The defect causes a deficiency of cortisol with an excess of pregnanetriol and androgens. In the severe (and less common) form, there is a sodium losing state after birth, which may be fatal. Male infants have normal external genitalia but females are virilised to some extent. In the milder form, salt losing is not apparent but androgen excess causes changes in childhood. The males develop partial precocious puberty, without testicular development. The females may have clitoral hypertrophy, rapid growth and early development of pubic and axillary hair but the breasts remain small and menstruation does not begin. Later male pattern hirsutes may appear.

C-11β hydroxylase deficiency. This defect involves the final steps of cortisol and aldosterone synthesis. Its severity is variable and the plasma cortisol may be normal but there is androgen and deoxycorticosterone excess causing virilisation and hypertension.

Diagnosis of the adrenogenital syndromes

A particular problem arises in the neonate. The extent of the virilisation of the external genitalia in the female ranges from clitoral hypertrophy to complete fusion of the labia and apparent hypospadias.

In the first 48 hours of life biochemical diagnosis is unreliable. Thereafter, for a time, plasma 17-α-hydroxyprogesterone may be the best test. After about eight days the urinary oxygenation index may be used. In some instances special biochemical tests are needed to determine the precise enzyme defect. Differentiation has to be made from true and pseudo hermaphroditism—chromosome analysis is necessary.

In older children, differentiation from true precocious puberty and virilising tumours of the ovary and adrenal is required.

Treatment

In the salt losing type, urgent treatment with corticosteroids and saline is life saving. Later, treatment is continued with hydrocortisone or prednisolone which suppresses excess androgen production and permits normal puberty and gonadal functions to emerge. It is sometimes advised that most of the corticosteroid dose should be given at night to achieve maximal suppression of ACTH. Therapy must be continued indefinitely in the female to prevent virilisation but whether long-term treatment is needed by the male remains to be seen. Plastic surgery for the external genitalia may be needed.

Prognosis

Except in the most severe forms the response to treatment is good and fertility normal. Patients are at risk from inadequate stress response and extra corticosteroid may be needed, but life expectancy may prove to be normal.

Adrenal tumours

In addition to the adrenal tumours described in connection with Cushing's and Conn's syndromes other tumours may secrete androgens, producing virilisation in the female, or oestrogens causing feminisation in the male, and a return of uterine bleeding in the post-menopausal female.

Location

Most of them are small and their deep position makes them difficult to find. Computerised tomography is the best method currently available for preoperative localisation but pyelography with tomography and angiography may succeed.

Hirsuitism and virilisation

In men this change is very rare and obviously difficult to identify—it is caused by a tumour secreting androgens. In women the problem is common but it is important to distinguish between hirsutism alone and the virilising syndromes.

Normal hair

The human is a hairy mammal and all the skin has hair follicles except the palms, soles and eyelids. The hair follicles are initially of the villus form, being relatively small and producing hairs which are short, thin, soft and pale. All follicles have the capacity to convert into the so-called 'terminal' form in which the follicle is bigger and produces hair which is longer, thicker, stiffer and usually darker. This conversion occurs on the scalp and eyebrows before or soon after birth. The next change is at puberty when a combination of adrenal, ovarian and testicular androgens induces a change to terminal hair in the axillae and lower pubic area. Later, in most women hair conversion occurs on the lower legs and, in some women, on the forearms. Normally, no further change occurs in the female until the menopause when some growth of teminal hair on the upper lip and chin is common and this persists into old age. The higher levels of androgens in late male puberty cause terminal hair to form in the typical areas of male hirsutes; the beard, lower abdomen, chest, arms and thighs. The typical male frontal baldness which progresses throughout adult life is thought to require a combination of a genetic factor and high androgens. It is presumed that the typical male sexual hair develops in areas where the follicles require a high level of androgens to undergo conversion. Once the conversion has taken place, reversal to the villus form is slow and uncertain. The term 'adrenarche' is sometimes used to indicate the time at about puberty when adrenal androgens increase and some sexual hair appears even in the absence of gonadal function.

Simple (idiopathic) hirsutism

The extent of terminal facial and body hair in normal women is variable. There are racial differences and women of Asiatic or Southern European origin have lower head hair lines and more body hair than Northern Europeans. Also, there is a cultural element in what is accepted as normal. (Fig. 9.4).

Clinical features. Obvious extra hair growth is likely to cause distress both because of the cosmetic effect and the unfounded fear that there will be a change of sex. The hair conversion begins to appear usually

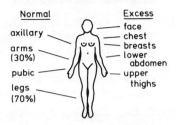

FIG. 9.4. The distribution of normal and 'excess' female hair. In normal women 30% have hair on the forearms and 70% have hair on their legs.

between puberty and the age of 20 years. It tends to increase slowly but usually this stops by the age of 35. The severity and distribution is variable. On the face the upper lip and chin are particularly affected. The hair on the forearms increase, long hair grows on and between the breasts and the pubic hair extends on to the upper thighs and up the anterior abdominal wall (the so-called 'male escutcheon'). The skin tends to be rather greasy and acne may appear. The menses and fertility may be normal but many of the patients have irregular periods and reduced fertility. The general health, blood pressure, breasts and clitoris are all normal.

Aetiology. It is not certain whether this is an intrinsic fault (e.g. increased sensitivity to androgen) in the hair follicles. Bio-chemical changes are slight but usually the plasma testosterone and perhaps other androgens are at the upper limit of the normal female range or slightly above it. It is debatable whether the androgens come from the adrenal or the ovary, or both.

Diagnosis. The large majority of women with excess hair have simple hirsutism. If there is no clitoral hypertrophy and the menses are regular (particularly if ovulation is occurring) it is most unlikely that any other endocrine disorder is present and complex investigations are not indicated. Nearly all other hirsute women have the polycystic ovary syndrome and this may require investigation particularly if fertility is desired. Plasma testosterone measurement is a satisfactory screening test in hirsutism to exclude the rare disorders of tumour or enzyme defect.

Treatment. This should include reassurance about the benign nature of the condition coupled with practical advice. It is of course the facial hair which causes most distress and *electrolysis* is probably the best local treatment. This involves passing an electric current through individual hair follicles, applying diathermy to the follicles, or, perhaps in the future, passing current down the individual hairs. Prolonged treatment may be needed as more hairs convert to the terminal form. It is tedious, expensive, rather uncomfortable and expert treatment is required, but it is the only safe way of destroying hair without scarring. Shaving is a cheap and effective alternative but few patients will adopt it. Depilatory creams, bleaches and heavy layers of cosmetics are useful also.

Three medical treatments are currently available. *Cyproterone acetate* is an anti-androgen which has been used extensively in some countries. It must be combined with oestrogen to ensure that conception does not take place during treatment because of possible teratogenic effects. A possible regime is cyproterone acetate 50 mg per day on days 5–14 of the cycle with ethinyl oestradiol 50 mg per day on days 5–21 of the cycle. *Oral contraceptives* with a relatively high oestrogen content will sometimes help, presumably by suppressing ovarian androgen production in those patients in whom the androgen is of ovarian origin. Alternatively, small doses of *prednisolone* may be used to suppress adrenal androgen production. The benefits of these treatments are slight and persist only while the therapies are continued. In view of this and their possible hazards in long-term use they cannot be recommended for this purpose.

Prognosis. The natural history of simple hirsutism is not clear but the impression is that the excess body hair does not spread much after 35 years of age and tends to regress after the menopause.

Virilising syndromes
In these conditions increasing hirsutism is accompanied by evidence of androgenic activity elsewhere with amenorrhoea, clitoral hypertrophy uterine atrophy and breast atrophy. Sometimes frontal balding occurs.

Differential diagnosis. The polycystic ovary syndrome should be considered although usually the virilisation in that condition is slight (see Chapter 12 for details). Other causes are Cushing's syndrome, adrenal adenoma or carcinoma, arrhenoblastoma of the ovary and late-onset adrenogenital syndrome. The pattern of steroid hormones in plasma and urine with stimulation and suppression may be needed to make the diagnosis but laparotomy may be unavoidable.

Hyperaldosteronism

Primary aldosteronism (Conn's syndrome)
This condition occurs most commonly in middle-aged women and is due to autonomous hypersecretion of aldosterone. The presenting feature is nearly always hypertension which will appear to be 'essential' and relatively benign, although headache may be prominent. Oedema is rare. The most important associated feature is persistent hypokalaemia (< 3·0 mmol/l) in the absence of any obvious cause such as diuretic administration or vomiting. Sometimes the patient has symptoms due to the hypokalaemia affecting the kidneys or neuromuscular system producing polyuria, nocturia, paraesthesiae, episodic hyporeflexic muscle weakness or paralysis.

Aetiology. Between half and three quarters of the patients have a small solitary adrenal adenoma with a typical yellow cut surface. The other patients have micro- or macro-nodular adrenocortical hyperplasia. The pathological features are due to hypertension or hypokalaemia.

Diagnosis. The unprovoked hypokalaemia is the most important feature; normokalaemic Conn's syndrome is very rare. The diagnosis is established by the demonstration of inappropriately high levels of aldosterone under strictly controlled conditions (see assessment of adrenocortical function above) with low plasma renin. At present, adenoma cannot be differentiated reliably from hyperplasia although various methods are being tried. The main problem is to differentiate this rare disease from the very common essential hypertension. Screening of plasma potassium levels is the best guide at present.

Treatment. Spironolactone, an aldosterone antagonist, reverses all the features of aldosteronism. This may be used as a diagnostic test, in preparation for surgery and as long-term treatment if operation is refused or contraindicated. If an adenoma is present it should be removed.

Secondary aldosteronism
This arises in any of the many circumstances causing a persistent stimulation of the secretion of renin. The clinical features and treatment are those of the primary condition and measurement of aldosterone is rarely needed. Secondary aldosteronism occurs also in the very rare conditions with a primary increase of renin secretion. These are due to hyperplasia of the juxta-glomerular cells in the kidney (Bartter's syndrome) or a tumour derived from the same cells.

Adrenocortical insufficiency

This relatively uncommon condition may be acute or chronic, and primary or secondary.

Acute adrenocortical insufficiency (adrenal crisis)
This is due to a sudden absolute or relative lack of cortisol associated with an intercurrent illness or stress. The clinical features are determined at first by the underlying condition followed by a general deterioration and perhaps headache, nausea, vomiting, diarrhoea and hypotension going on to shock and death. The adrenal damage may occur, due presumably to bacterial toxins, in severe infections. In septicaemia, particularly meningococcal, there may be bilateral adrenal haemorrhage associated with multiple haemorrhages elsewhere, particularly in the skin (Waterhouse–Friderichson syndrome). Massive adrenal haemorrhage may occur in the newborn, particularly after birth trauma. Alternatively, acute adrenal insufficiency may occur under any additional stress, even a mild infection, in a patient whose adrenal responsiveness is reduced either by pre-existing adrenal damage of any kind or a failure of ACTH response caused by pituitary damage or corticosteroid therapy (see below). Now that treatment with systemic corticosteroids and ACTH is so widely used the latter cause of insufficiency is the commonest.

Diagnosis. Usually the situation is urgent and diagnosis has to be made on clinical grounds to guide immediate treatment. It is desirable to use the schedule below to confirm the diagnosis as this will help later management.

Treatment. Blood is taken for cortisol assay. An intravenous infusion of one litre of normal saline per hour is begun and to each litre is added:

    Dexamethasone sodium phosphate 4 mg
    Aqueous tetracosactrin   250 μg

After an hour further blood is taken for cortisol assay. This regime achieves effective treatment while the cortisol assays will confirm the clinical diagnosis and assess adrenal responsiveness. During the following hours treatment should include more saline and corticosteroid as necessary, intravenous glucose and the treatment of any precipitating condition. Alternatively, intravenous hydrocortisone may be given with the saline but this precludes simultaneous testing. Long-term therapy will depend on circumstances and subsequent assessment.

Primary chronic adrenocortical insufficiency (Addison's disease)

Clinical features. The presentation is variable depending on the rapidity and degree of adrenal destruction. Onset is usually in middle-aged persons of either sex. The disease is slowly progressive over months or years with non-specific complaints of lassitude, weakness, anorexia, nausea and weight loss. There may be vomiting and abdominal pain; symptoms of hypoglycaemia and postural hypotension may occur. The presentation may be with an adrenal crisis from sudden stress. Depression or psychosis are not uncommon.

On examination, the patient is likely to be thin, weak and hypotensive. Pigmentation is the most striking feature. This is due to increased melanin and affects the skin generally with extra pigment in recent scars, pressure zones under straps and belts, palmar creases, the areolae and perineum, and areas exposed to sunlight. Dark freckles may appear and occasionally vitiligo. There may be patchy slate-grey pigmentation on the mucosa of cheeks, gums and lips. This buccal pigmentation may be seen in normal persons with black skin. The axillary hair is sparse, particularly in women, but usually ovarian function is normal.

Pathology. The illness is due to a lack of corticosteroid action but the relative importance of gluco- and mineralo-corticoid deficiency in producing symptoms is uncertain. The lack of aldosterone tends to cause sodium loss and potassium retention; blood glucose tends to be low.

The pigmentation is due to excess secretion of ACTH induced by the low level of plasma cortisol. The aetiology is 'idiopathic' or, rarely now, tuberculous. An auto-immune process is proposed for the former because usually autoantibodies are present, there is a clinical correlation with other presumed autoimmune endocrine conditions and the histology of the adrenal gland is reminiscent of that in lymphadenoid goitre. Very rarely other processes such as secondary neoplasm and granulomas may destroy the adrenal gland.

Diagnosis. This depends on the demonstration of a lack of adrenocortical response to ACTH (see above). The level of plasma cortisol is likely to be low and the diurnal rhythm lost but an adrenal crisis may occur in the presence of normal basal steroid levels with a failure of response to stress, so normal levels do not necessarily exclude the diagnosis. A raised level of plasma ACTH is confirmatory. Plasma electrolytes are unreliable in diagnosis. Adrenal calcification shown on radiographs indicates tuberculosis.

Treatment. The administration of hydrocortisone is the main therapy. An initial high dose may be helpful but for the long-term the correct dose is about 20 mg in the morning and 10 mg in the evening by mouth to reproduce the normal production rate and rhythm. Some additional mineralocorticoid is needed and usually fludrocortisone 100 μg each morning is suitable. Adjustments of dose may be needed to secure normal well being, blood pressure and body weight without oedema.

It is important to emphasise to the patient that the disability is permanent and that continuous treatment is essential, irrespective of other circumstances and drugs, with increased corticosteroid at times of stress. The patient must carry a 'steroid' card at all times.

Secondary adrenocortical insufficiency

In the chronic form this is part of the syndrome of anterior pituitary failure. Responsiveness to ACTH is retained but may be sluggish due to adrenal atrophy.

The acute form occurs when stress response fails in pituitary disease or after corticosteroid therapy (see below).

Treatment with corticosteroids and ACTH

It is necessary to distinguish *replacement* treatment, to correct a deficiency, from the administration of larger amounts which uses the *pharmacological* properties of the corticosteroids.

Replacement
In theory, ACTH could be given to patients with hypopituitarism to maintain adrenal function but the injections are inconvenient so that replacement treatment for primary or secondary adrenal lack is by oral corticosteroids. Hydrocortisone is preferable because it is the natural steroid but cortisone acetate is satisfactory despite the need for it to be deacetylated and then converted to cortisol in the liver. The details are given above in connection with chronic adrenocortical insufficiency. The same hydrocortisone regime is suitable in hypopituitarism but usually additional mineralocorticoid is not required. There are no undesirable side-effects of replacement corticosteroid therapy and the only hazard is the lack of stress response due to the primary condition.

Pharmacological
The applications of this therapy are far too numerous to discuss. Doses must be adjusted to circumstances. Treatment with ACTH, natural or

synthetic, produces its effect as a result of increased secretion of adrenocortical steroids which consists mostly of a 50:50 mixture of cortisol and DHA. There is no conclusive evidence that the latter confers any particular benefits and the former may cause difficulties because of its mineralocorticoid effect. The adrenal response to ACTH is variable so the dose required is unpredictable and the medication has to be injected. Despite these disadvantanges ACTH treatment is recommended by some clinicians for certain conditions including juvenile asthma, ulcerative colitis, Bell's palsy and acute multiple sclerosis. With the possible exception of growth in juvenile asthma there is no good evidence that ACTH is ever superior to corticosteroid in treatment but the various features listed above make strict clinical comparisons impossible so that there is room for different opinions. Certainly ACTH therapy does not avoid corticosteroid side-effects nor suppression of the hypothalamic-pituitary-adrenocortical (HPAC) axis (see below).

Complications of corticosteroid therapy

High doses of steroids for a few days seem harmless but treatment prolonged for more than 2–3 weeks carries such grave risks that it should never be used without clear indication and then at the lowest possible dose to achieve the desired effect.

Complications are of three types:

Direct corticosteroid action. This causes the typical obesity, striae and moon face. The skin is thinned and bruises easily. Aseptic necrosis of bone may occur but more frequently osteoporosis is accelerated leading to vertebral collapse and pathological fractures. Diabetes may be made overt or more difficult to control. Sodium retention, oedema and hypertension may occur with ACTH or hydrocortisone. A psychosis may be produced.

Altered tissue response. The anti-inflammatory effect reduces tissue resistance so that tuberculosis may be reactivated and pyogenic infections fail to localise, leading to septicaemia. The clinical features of septic conditions may be masked by an absence of fever and inflammation; peritonitis may be masked. Viral and fungal infections have an increased frequency and severity.

Suppression of HPAC system. After some time, treatment with corticosteroids at doses above the physiological suppresses ACTH secretion and causes adrenocortical atrophy. The HPAC response to stress is lost. Treatment with ACTH causes adrenal hypertrophy rather than atrophy but is equally suppressive of ACTH release and therefore both forms of treatment prevent a normal HPAC response to stress and their withdrawal may cause an adrenal crisis. When treatment is withdrawn recovery of HPAC function may take many months.

Precautions

The risks can be reduced but not removed. The use of synthetic corticosteroids with little mineralocorticoid activity will largely avoid salt retention, oedema and hypertension. Complications are unlikely if the dose is kept below 10 mg prednisolone or its equivalent each day.

For a patient on corticosteroids or ACTH extra stress must be met by sufficient administered corticosteroid to mimic the normal response. If the usual dose is 20 mg prednisolone a day it is appropriate to double the dose at the outset of a major illness and then return to the previous dose over a few days depending on progress. To cover major surgery, hydrocortisone 100 mg in 1 litre of normal saline per 24 h is satisfactory and larger doses are rarely needed (although often given). Subsequently, an increased dose of the usual oral corticosteroid will be needed for a few days only. When the stress is more prolonged the supplement must match it. If the previous dose of corticosteroid was high then it is unlikely that any supplement will be needed. It is not certain what duration of corticosteroid or ACTH treatment will cause a lack of stress response with danger during withdrawal of the therapy. As a general guide, treatment for up to two weeks seems safe and can be withdrawn over 48 h. Longer periods of treatment must be assumed to have suppressed the HPAC system and treatment must be withdrawn slowly.

The regime for doing this varies depending on the nature and severity of the underlying disease and on the dose and duration of treatment—a relapse of the illness may interrupt the regime. If the treatment is withdrawn with large changes in dose, each change is likely to produce symptoms of general malaise or tiredness. This seems to be due at least in part to the withdrawal of the euphoriant effect of corticosteroids. At lower levels of dosage, too large a reduction may precipitate the so-called 'limp rag syndrome' which comprises nausea, tiredness and generalised aches and pains. Additional corticosteroid relieves the symptoms rapidly. The daily dose of prednisolone can be reduced by 5 mg every two weeks until it is down to 10 mg and then by 1 mg every 1–2 weeks until it is stopped. The 1 mg tablets of prednisolone are useful. Often this regime must be modified—it can be shortened if treatment has been for a few months only. Even slower changes may be needed after many years of treatment but probably there is no duration of treatment after which withdrawal is impossible. Levels of plasma cortisol can be used to monitor recovery. It is not certain that any particular timing of doses during the day is beneficial and ACTH is not indicated.

A particular problem arises in the patient who has had treatment with corticosteroids or ACTH in the past but not at present. Cortisol levels may be adequate for normal life but the response to stress may be still impaired and an adrenal crisis occur. Opinions differ as to how long this danger persists. A reasonable compromise seems to be three months for most patients but twelve months if treatment has been maintained at high doses for years. If time permits the stress response can be tested but usually the problem is an acute one and within the time limits suggested corticosteroids should be given during anaesthesia or severe illness.

ADRENAL MEDULLA

This consists of cords of polyhedral chromaffin cells and has a rich autonomic nerve supply—similar cells are present in many other parts of the body.

Physiology

The functions of the adrenal medulla and the sympathetic nervous system are closely related, particularly in the synthesis of the catecholamines. (Fig. 9.5). There are considerable stores of catecholamines

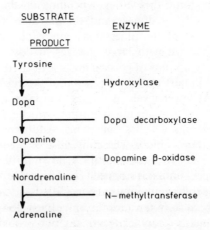

FIG. 9.5. The synthesis of the catecholamines.

in many tissues including the brain. Most of the adrenaline in the blood is released from the adrenal medulla but most of the noradrenaline comes from sympathetic nerve endings with only a small adrenal contribution. Catecholamine release is controlled by nerve impulses and responds to many drugs and stimuli but particularly stress including emotion, hypoglycaemia and trauma. In the circulation, catecholamines have a half life of a few minutes only, and are metabolised at many sites. Some catecholamine is taken up again by nervous tissue, some is methylated to form metanephrines and some is deaminated and then in part transformed to vanilmandelic acid (VMA). The metabolites are excreted in the urine, some of the metanephrines in the conjugated form.

The actions of catecholamines are many and vary with the amount present, the route of administration and pre-existing conditions. The actions of adrenaline and noradrenaline are qualititively similar but different in degree. Adrenaline acts on receptors causing smooth muscle contraction, and also, at other sites, β receptors causing smooth muscle relaxation. Noradrenaline acts mainly on α receptors. On the circulation the effect is generally stimulatory with increase in heart rate, blood pressure and arryhthmias. Oxygen consumption, plasma glucose and plasma free fatty acids are increased also but the detailed changes are highly complex. The significance of these effects in pathology generally and endocrinology in particular are uncertain and assessment of catecholamine function is rarely important in current practice.

Diseases of the adrenal medulla

No clinical condition due to adrenal medullary deficiency has been observed. Several different kinds of tumour may arise from medullary cells. Neuroblastoma is a highly malignant tumour which occurs in early childhood; some of its clinical features are due to hormone secretion. The only conditions producing disease due to catecholamine excess in adults are phaeochromocytoma and, perhaps, adrenal medullary hyperplasia.

Phaeochromocytoma

Clinical

The condition arises in young adults of either sex, and may be familial in association with neurofibromatosis or adenoma of other endocrine glands. The most common features are episodic headache, sweating, palpitations and hypertension. There is, however, considerable variability and the condition can mimic anxiety, hyperthyroidism, diabetes and spontaneous hypoglycaemia. Most importantly, episodic features may be absent and there is a sustained hypertension with the usual complications, indistinguishable at first from essential hypertension. On examination the patient is likely to be thin and to have lost weight. Hypertension may or may not be present. Features suggesting hyperthyroidism such as tremor, tachycardia and sweating may be found.

Pathology
Ninety per cent of phaeochromocytomas arise in the medulla but the others may occur anywhere in the sympathetic chain. Only about 10% are malignant and these may be bilateral.

The tumours are usually encapsulated and are grey-brown on section with patches of haemorrhage and necrosis. They are derived from chromaffin cells and stain accordingly.

Diagnosis
This depends on the demonstration of raised levels of catecholamines or their metabolites in the plasma or urine. The 24 h urine output of metanephrines is the usual test at present.

Further differentiation of adrenaline and noradrenaline excretion may be helpful as the latter is produced particularly by extra-medullary tumours. Blocking and stimulation tests have been largely discarded as they are unreliable and dangerous. Thyroid hormone levels are normal but biochemical diabetes may be present.

Treatment
This is by excision of the tumour(s). The procedure is dangerous because of the difficulty in stabilising the blood pressure before, during and after operation but successful anaesthetic techniques for this have been devised.

FURTHER READING

CHAN L. & O'MALLEY B. W. (1978). Steroid hormone action: Recent advances. *Annals of Internal Medicine,* **89,** 694.

CRAPO L. (1979). Cushings syndrome: A review of diagnostic tests. *Metabolism,* **28,** 955.

GIVENS J.R. (1976). Hirsutism and hyperandrogenism. *Advances in Internal Medicine,* **21,** 221.

NELSON D. (1980). *The Adrenal Cortex.* Saunders, London.

SCOTT H. *et al* (1976). Pheochromocytoma. *Annals of Surgery,* **183,** 587.

SKEGGS L.T. *et al* (1976). The biochemistry of the renin-angiotensin system and its role in hypertension. *American Journal of Medicine,* **60,** 737 (and following articles).

URBANIC R.G. & GEORGE J.M. (1981). Cushing's disease—18 years experience. *Medicine (Baltimore),* **60,** 14.

Chapter 10
Testis

ANATOMY

In the embryo the testes are formed on the posterior abdominal wall but soon move down to the deep inguinal ring. During the seventh month of gestation the testes migrate through the inguinal canals into the scrotum so that the spermatic cord, containing artery, vein and vas deferens follows the same course from scrotum to pelvis. The adult testis is about 4 cm long and 20–25 ml in volume. Histologically, the testes are composed mainly of seminiferous tubules. The basement membranes of the tubules are lined by two types of cell (i) spermatogonia from which spermatozoa are eventually derived, and (ii) Sertoli cells which act in a supporting (?nutrient) role to the germinal cells. The process of spermatogenesis within the germinal epithelium takes about ten weeks. It consists of the evolution of cells from spermatogonia through various types of spermatocytes and spermatids to mature spermatozoa which are discharged into the tubular lumen. There is a complex internal organisation within the germinal epithelium involving sequential changes of cell patterns and probable interaction of cells at various stages of development.

After discharge into the lumen, spermatozoa pass along finely coiled tubules and eventually into the epididymis which is a further long coiled tube leading into the vas deferens. Between the tubules lie groups of *Leydig* cells which secrete steroids, particularly testosterone.

In the fetal testis the Leydig cells develop, presumably stimulated by chorionic gonadotrophin, and the testosterone they produce is responsible in part for the differentiation of the male genital tract. The tubules are lined by undifferentiated cells and lack lumina. Soon after birth the Leydig cells regress. After the age of about five years the tubules develop gradually until both tubules and Leydig cells mature at puberty.

PHYSIOLOGY

Hormones of the testis

The Leydig cells contain the enzymes necessary to produce steroid hormones and several are synthesised, including oestrogen, but by far the most important in quantity and biological effect is testosterone. This is a C_{19}, OH–17 steroid (Fig. 10.1) and about 20 *u*mol are released (episodically) each day. It is likely that testosterone—at least for some tissues—has to be converted to dihydrotestosterone (DHT) (Fig. 10.1) before it exerts any biological activity. This occurs to some extent in

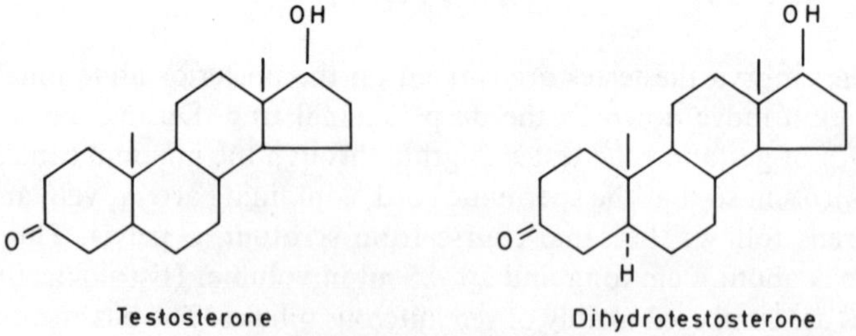

Testosterone   Dihydrotestosterone

FIG. 10. Structures of testosterone and dihydrotestosterone.

the circulation but mostly in the cytoplasm of the target organs. In addition, some DHT is released directly from the testis.

Control of Leydig cell function

These cells are stimulated by luteinising hormone (LH) from the anterior pituitary. This hormone used to be called 'interstitial cell stimulating hormone' in men but the hormone is identical in both sexes and it is now conventional to use the term LH. The release of LH is in turn suppressed by testosterone (see Chapter 8). Natural and synthetic oestrogens also will suppress LH release in men. There is a slight circadian rhythm of LH release and consequently the level of plasma testosterone rises during the night to a plateau during the middle of the day. It is doubtul whether the function of the germinal epithelium affects the levels of LH or testosterone.

Metabolism

Testosterone is carried in the plasma mostly bound to sex hormone binding globulin and albumin with about 2% in the free form. Testosterone is degraded, mostly in the liver and then conjugated to sulphate or glucuronides before excretion in the urine as a 17-oxosteroid. Only a small fraction of testosterone is converted to oestrogen but a major proportion of oestrogen in males is formed in this way.

Effects of androgens

The term 'androgen' is applied to steroids having actions similar to those of testosterone (Table 10.1).

TABLE 10.1 Actions of androgens

Fetal	Differentiation of male genitalia
Puberty	Linear growth spurt and epiphyseal fusion
	Masculine skeletal proportions (i.e. shoulders relatively wider than hips)
	Enlargement of larynx, breaking of voice
	Male hair pattern
	Enlargement of penis, scrotum with folds, and prostate
	Increased muscularity and strength
Psyche	Development of libido and potency
Metabolism	Protein anabolism (i.e. nitrogen retention)
In the female	Male hair distribution, laryngeal changes and clitoral hypertrophy. (Atrophy of breasts and uterus via gonadotrophin suppression and oestrogen lack)
Maintenance of masculinity	Once established, masculinity is maintained by minimal androgenic action

Synthetic anabolic steroids

Many synthetic steroids have been produced in an attempt to produce compounds with the protein anabolic effects of testosterone but without the androgenic effects. Some success has been achieved but the resulting compounds, sometimes called 'non-virilising androgens', have not found a major role in clinical practice.

Testicular tubular function

The maturation of the germinal epithelium at puberty requires the action of follicle stimulating hormone (FSH) from the anterior pituitary and a high concentration of testosterone—both are essential. It has been postulated that there is a feed-back loop via a non-steroid substance called '*inhibin*' secreted by the tubules which can suppress FSH. 'Inhibin' has not been isolated and the evidence for its existence is not conclusive. However, when damage to the germinal epithelium is severe, FSH secretion rises independently of changes in LH and testosterone showing that a control system does indeed exist.

PUBERTY

The initiation of puberty is not well-understood but it is suggested that during childhood the hypothalamus is relatively sensitive to androgen (including adrenal) and this suppresses the secretion of LH/FSH RH. As the hypothalamus matures this sensitivity diminishes. LH/FSH RH secretion begins, gonadotrophin secretion follows, then testicular maturation and the release of testosterone. Accordingly, the earliest stage of puberty is enlargement of the testicles. Beard growth is a late feature. The definition of the stages of puberty and the range of normal timing (Fig. 10.2) has been described by Tanner (see Further reading.) The assessment of testicular volume is done by comparison with an '*orchidometer*' which consists of a series of ovoid spheres ranging in volume from 2 to 25 ml.

AGEING

There is no doubt that there is a male climacteric ('menopause') but it is gradual, relative, more variable and lacks specific features compared to that in the female. Due to a slow primary testicular failure testosterone production falls gradually and variably after the age of forty.

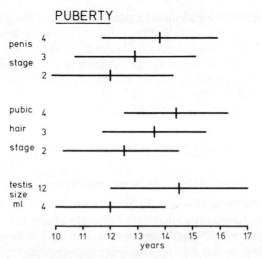

FIG. 10.2. The timing of male puberty. Each horizontal line includes 94% of all normals, i.e. 3% are earlier and 3% are later. Vertical lines show the age at which 50% of normal boys have reached that stage of development.

However, the levels of sex hormone binding globulin rise so that the level of plasma free testosterone falls substantially; by the age of seventy or eighty it is down to pre-pubertal levels. Levels of LH rise in response. There is a gradual loss of potency but fertility may be preserved into old age.

ASSESSMENT OF TESTICULAR FUNCTION

Hormonal

The measurement of plasma testosterone is the most useful test at present. A raised level of plasma LH indicates a primary testicular fault. Measurement of plasma testosterone after stimulation with human chorionic gonadotrophin (which acts like LH) may be used to test Leydig cell responsiveness. Neither testosterone nor gonadotrophin measurements will predict the future onset of puberty; they rise only as puberty progresses.

Tubules: seminal fluid examination (sperm count)

A fresh specimen of semen obtained by masturbation into a clean glass container is allowed to liquefy and the sperms counted within 1–2 h. A fresh smear is made to estimate the proportion of sperms with normal motility. Examination of sperm morphology and chemical analysis of semen may be done also. Various normal values for semen examination have been published, perhaps because individual specimens from the same man differ markedly. The volume is 2–6 ml and the sperm count usually over 60×10^6 ml but counts as low as 20×10^6 ml may be consistent with fertility. In general, the better the quality of the semen in all respects the greater the likelihood of conception.

DISEASES OF THE TESTES

Maldescent of the testes ('cryptorchidism')

At birth about 90% of testes are in the scrotum and most of the rest appear soon afterwards so that by the time of puberty only about 0.5% remain undescended, usually unilaterally. During childhood the testes may withdraw readily into the inguinal canal (pseudocryptorchidism.) It is likely that many maldescended testes are abnormal but only in a few instances can the aetiology be found.

Management is debatable and it is particularly difficult to decide at what age action should be taken. The following is a plausible scheme of management, but some clinicians would disagree:

1. Providing the external genitalia are normal otherwise, and the boy is of normal height, nothing should be done before the age of ten years. If there is doubt about the genitalia or if neither testicle can be displaced into the scrotum a chromosome analysis is indicated.
2. At the age of ten or at the onset of puberty, a course of human chorionic gonadotrophin (HCG) may be given (4000 units by injection, three times a week for three weeks.) If the testis descends it can be assumed that it will do so again later in puberty even if it retracts in the meantime.
3. If HCG has no effect, surgical exploration should be done. This permits the correction of a hernia if present, the identification of a truly ectopic testis and the securing of the testis in the scrotum (orchidopexy) if possible.
4. If maldescent is found after puberty it is said that the testes should be removed because of the risk of malignancy.

Testicular tumours

The majority of testicular tumours are malignant and few secrete hormones. Tumours containing choriocarcinoma secrete HCG, the findings of which in the urine is a useful marker. Leydig cell tumours may secrete androgens and cause precocious puberty but have little effect in adults. Rarely, a Leydig cell tumour secretes oestrogens and causes feminisation.

Primary hypogonadism

Testicular failure may affect the Leydig cells, the germinal tissue or both. Failure of Leydig cell function alone is recognised only in two circumstances, namely the slow decline with ageing (see above) and the failure of steroid production in some rare forms of the adrenogenital syndrome. The isolated failure of the germinal tissue causes infertility alone without other consequences and is discussed below.

Combined tubular and Leydig cell failure

There is considerable variation in the relative severity of damage to each component.

Clinical

The presentation will depend on the age at which testicular damage occurred. If it was early, puberty will not occur and unless there is a local defect such as maldescent, the problem comes to light only at that stage. Later, when adult, the patient usually presents a eunuchoid appearance, being of average height or above because growth continues until the middle twenties. The arms and legs are relatively long compared with the trunk so that the span is greater than the height and the pubis to heel distance is greater than the pubis to crown distance. Body fat varies but body contours tend to be feminine with relatively broad hips, and the musculature tends to be poor. Pubic and body hair is sparse and beard growth absent. The penis and scrotum are poorly developed and the testes small and firm. Bilateral gynaecomastia is common. Libido and potency are small or absent, and behaviour may be rather timid. The eunuchoid features are variable and occasionally Leydig cell function approaches normal, so that eunuchoid features are less marked. With rare exceptions the patients are infertile. If the testicular damage occurs after puberty the body form is normal and the secondary sexual characteristics are lost slowly over many years. Libido and potency may be remarkably well preserved.

Aetiology

Testicular agenesis (anorchia). In this rare condition only tiny hyalinised remnants of the testis can be found in the poorly developed scrotum.

Maldescent. Bilateral maldescent suggests a severe testicular defect either primary or secondary to the abnormal position of the testis. Unilateral maldescent is important also because often the other testis, although apparently normal, has diminished function particularly of the tubules.

Seminiferous tubule dysgenesis (Klinefelter's syndrome). Most patients with this condition have abnormal sex chromosomes, typically a 47 XXY with a chromatin positive buccal smear (see Chapter 11). Chromosome mosaics may occur. The incidence is about 1:600 male births. The degree of tubular and Leydig cell damage is variable and some patients seem normal males. There is an increased incidence of behaviour disorders and poor intelligence.

Associated congenital abnormalities. There are rare forms of hypo-gonadism due presumably to genetic faults and associated with other defects as in *dystrophia myotonia*, the *Laurence-Moon-Biedl* syndrome and *Reifenstein's* syndrome.

Acquired lesions

Bilateral torsion of the testes occurs in the presence of a congenital anomaly of the tunica vaginalis and may cause severe damage.

Bilateral orchitis occurs in many virus infections, but particularly in mumps. Usually, recovery is complete but if the orchitis is severe it may be followed by atrophy.

Miscellaneous. The testes may be damaged by radiation, cytotoxic drugs and iron deposition in haemochromatosis. There is damage also in cirrhosis, due perhaps to changes in steroid metabolism, and in para-plegia in which case the cause is obscure. In general the germinal epithelium is damaged more readily than the Leydig cells. Probably alcohol causes a direct depression of testicular function.

Diagnosis

The diagnosis of primary hypogonadism before puberty is impossible unless the testes are abnormal and can be confirmed only if there is a detectable chromosome fault. After puberty, the cause may be obvious from the history and physical examination. Measurement of plasma testosterone will establish the level of Leydig cell function. A raised plasma LH excludes secondary hypogonadism. A raised plasma FSH has the same significance but in addition indicates a severe defect of the germinal epithelium. Chromosome examination may be invaluable. Rarely, testicular biopsy may be necessary.

Treatment
Replacement androgen treatment for Leydig cell failure is adequate (see below). There is no useful treatment for primary damage to the germinal epithelium and correction of androgen deficiency does not help.

Secondary hypogonadism

The clinical features depend on whether the failure of gonadotrophin secretion is an isolated defect or part of a panhypopituitarism, and the age at which the defect occurs.

Pre-pubertal

Isolated gonadotrophin deficiency. This is a rare condition in which gonadotrophin secretion does not rise at the time of normal puberty but hypothalamic-pituitary function is normal otherwise. Conventionally, the patient has to reach the age of 18 before puberty is considered to have failed rather than just be delayed, but psychological pressures in patient or parents may make it impossible to wait that long. The condition may be familial and there may be associated congenital abnormalities. Anosmia may be present in which case the term *'Kallman's syndrome'* is used. Injections of LH/FSH RH causes secretion of gonadotrophin suggesting that the primary defect is in the hypothalamus. Treatment with HCG (4000 units by injection, three times a week) for several months will induce puberty but not fertility. Sometimes after one or more courses of treatment normal function develops. Otherwise, long-term androgen treatment is needed.

Panhypopituitarism. The gonadotrophin deficiency is a part of the condition which is characterised particularly by slow growth and/or short stature. There are many possible causes (see Chapter 8) but one of the commonest is a craniopharyngioma.

Post-pubertal

Isolated gonadotrophin deficiency in a previously normal adult male is rare but may cause gradual loss of secondary sexual characteristics, impotence and infertility. Androgen treatment will correct all these except the infertility.

Panhypopituitarism (see Chapter 8) causes a clinical picture which is dominated by adrenal and thyroid failure with the hypogonadism of relatively minor importance. Androgen treatment may be helpful but is not always essential; it may help to retard osteoporosis.

ANDROGEN REPLACEMENT TREATMENT

Testosterone itself is relatively inactive when taken orally. Methyl testosterone can be taken sub-lingually but may cause cholestatic jaundice. Fluoxymesterone (10–20 mg/day, orally) is safer but relatively ineffective and full replacement is difficult to achieve. The best treatment is intramuscular injections of testosterone esters in a dose of 50 mg per week or 250 mg each month. The response may be slow with a progressive effect, particularly on hair growth, over several years. The response in sexual function and mental state is excellent.

DELAYED PUBERTY

This is a relatively common problem and naturally of great concern to the boy and his parents.

Management
The first step is to compare the boy's age and stage of sexual development with normal data (see further reading and Fig. 10.2) and also the height with charts of normal growth (see Chaper 8). A general physical examination is essential. There is no way of predicting puberty so management has to be flexible. A possible strategy is:
1. If puberty is in fact *not* retarded (i.e. not later than the 3rd percentile) with normal height and physical examination, reassurance and continued observation are indicated.
2. If puberty is late but height normal, a primary testicular failure should be suspected and investigated with chromosome analysis and hormone assays. If investigations are negative further observation until age 18 or so may be advised, if acceptable psychologically, and then a course of HCG given. If there is no permanent benefit, puberty will have to be induced with androgens.
3. If puberty is late and height retarded the pituitary should be investigated.

If the tests are negative the condition is presumably 'constitutional' and prolonged observation may be the best treatment as many such boys eventually develop normally. Alternatively, puberty may be induced with androgens but this might reduce eventual height by causing early epiphyseal fusion.

Positive results of investigations may of course dictate management at any stage.

PRECOCIOUS PUBERTY (SEXUAL PRECOCITY)

There are two types, complete and partial.

Complete
This means a typical puberty with all the usual features (and in the usual order in most patients) through to sexual maturity but at an abnormally early age. In rare instances the condition is 'idiopathic' and the patient is eventually a normal adult. More commonly, precocious puberty in boys is due to organic cerebral disease, such as tumour, encephalitis or hydrocephalus. There is no generally accepted treatment but progestogens and antiandrogens have been tried.

Partial
This means incomplete puberty due to ectopic production of gonadotrophin or androgen. In the former case the puberty may be virtually normal but a tumour producing gonadotrophin is always malignant and shortly declares itself. Ectopic androgens may come from a Leydig cell tumour or the adrenogenital syndrome and produce virilisation without testicular development. Precocious puberty may of course be produced by the deliberate or inadvertent administration of hormones.

GYNAECOMASTIA

At puberty
Some enlargement of breast tissue occurs in many boys at puberty. They develop a tender sub-areolar plaque 1–2 cm in diameter which shrinks slowly and seldom persists for more than a few years. It is not uncommon for the breast enlargement to be greater and become obvious. The change may be unilateral and sometimes the nipple changes to the typical domed female type. It has been suggested that puberty gynaecomastia is due to a relative excess of oestrogen compared to androgen during mid-puberty, but the occurrence of unilateral gynaecomastia implies variation in tissue responsiveness also.

Management. Gynaecomastia causes great embarrassment and raises doubts about the boy's masculinity and future behaviour. Physical examination will determine whether puberty is normal otherwise. It is important to differentiate true gynaecomastia from the swellings due to fat seen in obese boys in whom no breast tissue can be felt. If puberty is satisfactory otherwise, investigation can be limited to a buccal smear for nuclear chromatin. If this is normal, strong reassurance to the boy and his parents is important. The breast tissue tends to shrink over several years but if desired it can be removed surgically with preservation of the nipples. There is no established medical treatment.

If the puberty or nuclear chromatin is suspect then full investigation is necessary as gynaecomastia is a common accompaniment of primary testicular damage.

Adult

In the adult, gynaecomastia can be due to many causes of which the following are probably the commonest:

  Primary testicular failure,
  Liver disease
  Drugs, particularly spironolactone, digoxin and phenothiazines
  Refeeding (i.e. restoration of nutrition after severe ilness)
  Carcinoma, particularly bronchial
  Endocrine disease, e.g. pituitary tumours, thyroid disease and acro-
    megaly
  Oestrogens—e.g. stilboestrol for prostatic cancer or from an oestro-
    gen secreting tumour
  Paraplegia and chest trauma.

Rarely, galactorrhoea may occur and suggests hyperprolactinaemia. Management comprises the search for and treatment of the underlying condition.

SIZE OF GENITALIA

Anxiety about underdevelopment of the genitalia may be expressed by parents of pre-pubertal boys or later as part of concern about delayed puberty or lack of sexual function. In the younger child the problem is due usually to obesity in which the penis is buried in the suprapubic fat and appears smaller than it really is. The penis may be measured and compared with tables of normality (see Further reading).

In the older patient, unless there is an obvious fault, the problem is likely to be one of unreasonable expectations and serious psychological problems may be involved. Androgen therapy will not help. The devices now advertised to increase penis size are probably harmless but do not appear to have been subjected to scientific evaluation.

IMPOTENCE

This is a lack of physical capability for erection and/or ejaculation and may or may not be accompanied by a lack of libido i.e. sexual interest or desire. Occasionally, ejaculation fails despite normal erection but this is usually a minor transient disorder due to fatigue or alcohol. The causes of impotence may be grouped under four headings:

Hypogonadism
Primary, or secondary, with a failure of potency due to androgen deficiency. A high level of plasma prolactin may cause impotence. If the fault arises before puberty sexual function is never established but with a later onset, potency may be lost before libido which is more a matter of habit. A similar situation occurs from an excess of endogenous oestrogen (from a tumour or cirrhosis of the liver) or therapy with oestrogens. There is a slow loss of potency, particularly in the speed and completeness of erection as a consequence of the male climacteric.

Drugs
Many antihypertensive drugs and some tranquillisers impair erection. Alcohol can have the same effect.

Neurological
Autonomic neuropathy (most commonly from diabetes) and damage to the nerve supply by pelvic surgery may prevent erection.

Psychogenic
This may be an isolated complaint or accompany mental illness, particularly depression. The isolated form may be selective and occur only with certain partners. There is likely to be a background of personal dysharmony.

Management
Physical causes should be sought by routine examination and history. An exploration of the patient's personal relationships and mental state is helpful. If there is doubt about testicular function the measurement

of plasma testosterone will help but the level may be slightly reduced in psychogenic impotence. Hyperprolactinaemia may be sought.

Treatment should remove possible underlying factors such as drugs and also help preceding psychiatric illness. If plasma testosterone is normal, androgen therapy is unlikely to help but it is harmless and the patient may expect it. There is no treatment for the neurological types and usually the defect is permanent.

The treatment of isolated psychogenic impotence has been improved by the introduction of behavioural methods of the Masters and Johnson type but usually hormones are unhelpful.

INFERTILITY

Between 10% and 15% of marriages are infertile. The defect is about equally likely in either sex so that, unless there is some obvious cause, both partners should be investigated.

Aetiology

The causes of male infertility are poorly understood and in about half the patients no fault can be found. Only a small minority have a major disorder such as hypopituitarism or Klinefelter's syndrome. A rather larger number have varicocele or vas obstruction. The remainder have a primary defect of the germinal epithelium, the cause of which is unknown, although chromosomal faults in the germ cells may be important.

Classification of germinal epithelium defects in infertility
There is no generally agreed classification but the following seems helpful. In all types the Leydig cells appear normal or increased in number, the latter perhaps due to diminished tubular mass. The basement membrane of the tubules may be thickened.

Germinal cell aplasia (Sertoli-cell-only syndrome.) The most severe form of tubular epithelium damage. The germ cells are virtually absent leaving only the Sertoli cells, hence the alternative name.

Germinal cell hypoplasia. Diminished activity of the germinal epithelium, possibly an earlier stage of the 'aplasia' condition.

Maturation arrest. Germ cell evolution seems to be normal up to a certain stage, usually primary spermatocytes or spermatids, but the later stages are not present.

Obstruction. The germinal epithelium seems normal except for sloughing and vacuolisation but the tubules are dilated.

Management

History. Duration of infertility. It is reasonable to postpone investigations until a year has elapsed. Enquire as to the normality and frequency of intercourse and whether it has been concentrated at the time of ovulation. A spermicide may have been used inadvertently, perhaps as a lubricant. A history suggesting testicular damage, e.g. delayed puberty, maldescent, orchitis, etc, may be found.

Examination. The testicles should be examined and their size estimated. Varicocele (usually on the left side) should be sought by examining the scrotum with the patient standing. General examination should try to confirm normal masculine development and seek evidence of endocrinopathy, particularly hypopituitarism and hypothyroidism.

Investigation. A sperm count is essential.

Review
At this stage the situation should be reviewed. If all is normal, particularly the sperm count, further investigation of the man should be postponed for six to twelve months for further attempts at conception. If this is unsuccessful or if the initial sperm count is low, further investigation is indicated.

Hormone assay. For plasma testosterone and FSH. Low testosterone and high gonadotrophin suggests a severe primary testicular defect and chromosome examination is necessary. If testosterone is normal but FSH high, there is likely to be severe primary damage of the germinal epithelium. If testosterone and FSH are both low, a pituitary fault is likely and further investigation needed.

Testicular biopsy. This is not a routine test. It is unlikely to be helpful if there is azoospermia and raised FSH, or if a pituitary defect is present. It may be helpful, particularly in prognosis, if there is azoospermia with normal hormone levels.

Treatment
The prospects for treatment of male infertility are bad. Ligation of a varicocele is conventional practice but its value is now questioned. There is no evidence that androgen therapy is of benefit. If there is oligospermia, concentration of semen and artificial insemination has been used. Azoospermia with normal spermatogenesis in the biopsy suggests vas obstruction; this may be defined by vasography and reconstructive operations have been attempted but with little success. In hypogonadotrophic infertility treatment with gonadotrophins has been successful in a very few patients.

Treatment of germinal cell aplasia, hypoplasia and maturation arrest has been unsuccessful and the patient should be told that further treatment is futile.

FURTHER READING

BURGER H. & de KRETSER D. (Eds) (1981). *The Testis*. Raven Press, New York.

FONKALSRUD E.W. & MENGEL W. (Eds) (1981). *The Undescended Testis*. Year Book Medical Publishers, Chicago.

FOREST M.G. *et al* (1976). Hypothalamic-pituitary gonadal relationships in man from birth to puberty. *Clinical Endocrinology*, **5**, 557.

HSUEH W.A. *et al* (1978). Endocrine features of Klinefelter's syndrome. *Medicine* (Baltimore), **57**, 447.

LEE P.A. *et al* (1978). Micropenis. I. Criteria, etiologies and classification. *The Johns Hopkins Medical Journal, 146*, 156.

ODELL W.D. SWERDLOFF R.S. (1978). Abnormalities of gonadal function in man. *Clinical Endocrinology*, **8**, 149.

PHILIP E.E. & CARRUTHERS G.B. (Eds) (1981). *Infertility*. Heinemann, London.

STEINBERGER E. (1978). The etiology and pathophysiology of testicular dysfunction in man. *Fertility and Sterility*, **29**, 481.

TANNER J.M. (1962) *Growth at Adolescence* (2nd Edition). Blackwell Scientific Publications, Oxford.

(Excellent charts containing the normal ranges for the stages of puberty from Tanner and Marshall are available from Creaseys of Hertford Ltd, Castlemead, Hertfordshire.)

Chapter 11
Disorders of Sex Differentiation

It is not uncommon for individuals to have such mental or physical characteristics that they cannot be said with confidence to be male or female. There is no simple criterion of gender and for an individual it may be helpful to describe their sex under several characteristics, i.e. genetic form (genotype), general habitus (phenotype), gonads, internal genitalia, external genitalia, hormones and gender role. In the intersexual states these characteristics are more or less discordant. Their classification here is much abbreviated and many rare forms have been omitted.

Because they are dealt with elsewhere in the text this discussion *excludes*:

1. Phenotypic males with abnormal chromosomes (Klinefelter's syndrome— Chapter 10).
2. Phenotypic females with abnormal chromosomes (Turner's syndrome— Chapter 12).
3. Masculinising syndromes in previously normal females (Chapter 12).
4. Feminising syndromes in previously normal males (Chapter 12).

In the normal six week-old human fetus there are primitive gonads of indeterminate sex. Shortly afterwards the sex determining genes in the X and Y chromosomes may cause a differentiation of the gonads into testes. If the genetic constitution is female however, the undifferentiated gonad persists and ovarian structures do not appear until the twelfth week.

By eight weeks the fetus contains both the müllerian ducts, which can develop into female internal genitalia, and the wolffian ducts which can develop into male internal genitalia. During the following month one pair of ducts complete their development while the alternative involutes. If ovaries are present, or no gonads at all, it is the female structures which are formed. If a testis is present, it causes male development on that side. The stimulation of the wolffian ducts is due to androgen from the testis but the involution of the müllerian ducts is caused by an unidentified nonsteroidal substance which the testis secretes also.

The eight week-old fetus has indeterminate external genitalia which can differentiate into male or female structures. If ovaries are present, or no gonads, normal female development occurs without hormonal stimulus. Androgen from the testes causes the external genitalia to differentiate into the male form. Exogenous androgen can have the same effect. Intermediate levels of androgenic stimulation in both sexes produce intermediate external genitalia.

In general, inherent sexual differentiation is directed into the female pattern unless specifically deflected. The genetic control is through the gonads and particularly by the early development of the testes. There is no evidence of fetal sexual differentiation in the human hypothalamus or brain.

HERMAPHRODITISM

This term is derived from Greek mythology. The god Hermaphroditus was born of Hermes and Aphrodite (the archetypal male and female) and had some of the physical characteristics of both sexes. In Greco-Roman art the god is depicted usually as having a female head and breasts with male genitalia suggesting that examples of Klinefelter's syndrome may have been the origin of the legend. 'Hermaphroditism' as a technical term is applied to individuals who have both testicular and ovarian tissue. 'Pseudohermaphroditism' is the term applied to those in whom the gonads and external genitalia are discordant.

Ambiguous genitalia

These arise as a result of abnormal development of the external genitalia in the fetus with variation mainly in the extent of fusion of the labial folds, the position of the urethra and the size of the phallus. Many variants have been recorded.

True hermaphroditism

This extremely rare condition is characterised by the presence of gonads containing both ovarian and testicular tissue (ovotestis) or one testis with one ovary. The phenotype can vary from almost normal male to normal female; the karyotype is variable also.

Male pseudohermaphroditism

Non-familial. These patients have testes, usually in the abdomen, variable external genitalia, no uterus and usually a 46 XY karyotype although some are mosaics.

Familial. This variety is also termed the 'testicular feminisation' syndrome. (See Chapter 13-primary amenorrhoea.)

Female pseudohermaphroditism

This is usually due to the adrenogenital syndrome in otherwise normal females (46 XX). Enzyme defects cause excess androgen production from the adrenal which leads to a variable degree of virilisation of external genitalia of the fetus (see Chapter 9). Most of the few remaining patients have been influenced by androgens given to or produced by their mother during pregnancy, but rarely no cause can be found.

EXAMINATION OF CHROMOSOMES AND CHROMATIN

Chromosomes

A cell culture is prepared, usually of blood leucocytes. Substances are added to stimulate cell division and then to arrest dividing nuclei in the metaphase. The chromosomes are photographed and classified in a standard format to produce a 'karyotype'. Various staining techniques may be used to provide further information. In normal persons there are 23 pairs of chromosomes; one pair are the sex chromosomes, designated XX (female) or XY (male). The normal female karyotype is therefore 46 XX and the normal male 46 XY. Normally, all somatic cells have the same karyotype but sometimes two or more cell lines with different karyotypes may be present. This is called a 'mosaic' and may lead to sex chromatin being present in a proportion of cells intermediate between the normal male and normal female.

Only variations in the sex chromosomes are relevant to sex differentiation. Many types have now been recorded; a few of the best known are shown in Table 11.1. Sex chromosome patterns as currently reported are not necessarily specific to the clinical syndromes.

TABLE 11.1. Some sex chromosome patterns

Type	Frequency	Consequences
45 X	1:3000	Turner's syndrome
46 XX	—	Normal female
47 XXX	1:1600	Uncertain
46 XY	—	Normal male
47 XXY	1:600	Klinefelter's syndrome
47 XYY	1:1100	Excessive height

Nuclear chromatin examination. This is carried out conveniently on squamous cells scraped from the inside of the cheek (a buccal smear). The deposit is spread on a slide, fixed and stained. On microscopy of a smear from a normal female, 20% to 50% of the cells show a single distinctive dark dot just under the nuclear membrane. The dot is called the sex chromatin or 'Barr' body and consists of chromatin from an X chromosome. The number of Barr bodies present is always one less than the number of X chromosomes because, according to the 'Lyon' hypothesis, only one chromosome is genetically active. Other X chromosomes complete their DNA synthesis late in the interphase and form Barr bodies. Thus normal male cells (46 XY) never contain Barr bodies, normal female cells (46 XX) contain one Barr body, and in a woman with a 47 XXX karyotype two Barr bodies would be present. The Lyon hypothesis of X chromosome inactivation has profound implications for the genetics of sex differentiation and sex linkage.

Nuclear chromatin examination is a simple test. It is useful in screening to identify those patients in whom the more complex chromosome examination is indicated.

MANAGEMENT OF THE PATIENT OF UNCERTAIN PHYSICAL SEX

There are three stages:

1. Diagnosis
2. Assignment of gender
3. Treatment.

There are great advantages if these problems are dealt with at the earliest possible moment so that the patient presents usually as a new-born child with ambiguous genitalia. The parents must be told at once and the appropriate investigations carried out. Hormone assays will detect congenital adrenal hyperplasia, chromosome studies are essential and biopsy of the gonads, perhaps by laparotomy, may be needed. The assignment of gender is not necessarily obvious. The potential of the existing external genitalia is probably the most important single factor as it is much easier to construct female genitalia surgically, than male. The parents' cooperation in the decision is essential. Once gender assignment has been made, the early stage of surgical correction can be carried out and any inappropriate gonad removed. The infant can be named and registered appropriately. Later, further surgery may be needed and probably hormone replacement treatment at puberty.

In the older patient, the problem is likely to be far more difficult and account must be taken of the person's sex, of rearing, and personal wishes. At all ages, much mental support of the patients and relations may be needed.

DISORDERS OF MENTAL SEXUAL DIFFERENTIATION

What are now generally accepted as normal variants of sexual behaviour particularly homosexuality, lesbianism and fetishism, do not have an endocrinological basis and do not require hormone therapy.

Gender transfer (trans-sexualism)

This is a more serious problem, which is not as rare as once supposed. Contrary to earlier reports, it is probable that both sexes are equally likely to be affected. The patients are, so far as can be determined, physically entirely normal males or females in all respects. They are seized by an overwhelming conviction that they are in fact of the opposite sex to their physical constitution. This belief appears early in childhood, is not accompanied by any features of mental illness and appears to be totally unaltered by any kind of argument or psychiatric treatment. It is uncertain whether this condition has an organic basis, related perhaps to the hormonal environment *in utero* or is a psychological disorder, related to the emotional environment during infancy and childhood.

Management
An unknown proportion of these individuals refuse to accept their

situation and wish to 'pass', i.e. to change their names, clothes and behaviour to what they believe to be their correct gender. In the UK, if supported by medical evidence, they may change their sex of registration for National Insurance and employment purposes but not with the Registrar General. They seek medical help also to convert their physical form to that of the opposite sex. There is an ethical dilemma for the doctor in deciding how far to assist in this change but some surgeons are prepared to operate. The removal of breasts, uterus and male external genitalia are straight-forward enough as surgical procedures and a satisfactory vagina can be made, but the problems of constructing a workable penis have not yet been overcome. Hormone treatment may be requested to produce the desired secondary sexual characteristics. It may be difficult to find a relatively safe dose that satisfies the patient; the long-term consequences are unknown.

FURTHER READING

DEWHURST C.J. (1975). The aetiology and management of intersexuality. *Clinical Endocrinology*, **4**, 625.

JONES H.W. & SCOTT W.W. (1971). *Hermaphroditism, Genital Anomalies and Related Endocrine Disorders* (2nd edition). Williams and Wilkins, Baltimore.

SIMPSON J.L. (1976). *Disorders of Sexual Differentiation*. Academic Press, London.

WACHTEL S.S. (1979). The genetics of intersexuality: clinical and theoretic perspectives. *Obstetrics and Gynaecology*, **54**, 671.

Chapter 12
Ovary

ANATOMY

The adult ovaries weigh about 7 g each and measure $3 \times 2 \times 1$ cm; they are attached by the ovarian ligaments to the backs of the broad ligaments. Microscopically, the ovary has a capsule of connective tissue, the tunica albuginea, and then a cortex containing the follicles embedded in a supportive tissue called the stroma.

PHYSIOLOGY

Hormones

The ovary produces three kinds of steroids—oestrogens, androgens and progesterone. The cellular origins of the hormones are mixed and there is no ovarian equivalent of the Leydig cell. Oestrogens are produced by several cell types but particularly the theca cells; androgens produced by thecal cells are aromatised by the granulosa cells. The

179

principal oestrogen is oestradiol (Fig. 12.1) but oestrone is present in the plasma also, in similar concentration. Some oestrone is released by the ovary, some is formed by conversion from oestradiol and some by conversion from other steroids. Progesterone (Fig. 12.1) is secreted mainly by the corpus luteum. The androgens, particularly testosterone, may be produced by cells at the ovarian hilum. The secretion of testosterone is about 5% of that from the testes.

The secretion of the ovarian hormones is under the control of the anterior pituitary gonadotrophins with considerable fluctuations during the menstrual cycle (see Chapter 13). Oestradiol in the plasma is bound less well than testosterone to sex hormone binding globulin but better than testosterone to albumin. The metabolism of oestradiol is principally by the liver to a relatively inactive compound oestriol which is conjugated with glucuronic acid and excreted in the urine. Progesterone is converted to pregnanediol and excreted in the urine also as a glucuronide.

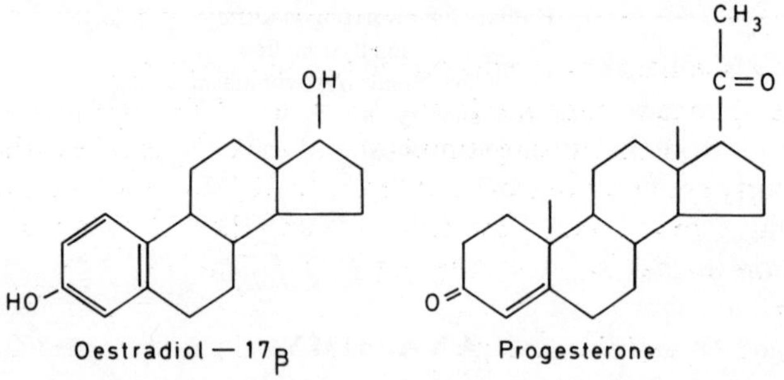

FIG. 12.1. The structures of oestradiol and progesterone.

Action of oestrogens
These are given in Table 12.1. The actions of synthetic oestrogens such as mestranol are largely the same as those of 'natural' oestrogens both animal and human, but the activity of stilboestrol *in utero* is an exception. The effects of oestrogens on the psyche are poorly understood and their importance for libido and the capacity for orgasm is uncertain. The hazards of oestrogens when used as pharmacological agents, e.g. in oral contraceptives, are discussed in Chapter 13.

NORMAL PUBERTY

It is suggested that during childhood the hypothalamus is relatively sensitive to sex steroids, presumably including adrenal androgen.

7

TABLE 12.1 Physiological actions of oestrogens

Puberty	—	Linear growth spurt and epiphyseal fusion. Broadening of pelvis
		Growth of pubic and axillary hair
		Breast and nipple enlargement
		Maturation of external genitalia
		Initiation and maintenance of menstruation (with progesterone)
		Increase in subcutaneous fat
Psyche	—	Supports libido (?)
Metabolism	—	May cause salt and water retention
Maintenance	—	Maintains vaginal mucosa and secretion, uterus and breast tissue
		? Maintains skeletal bulk and skin texture
		? Protects against arterial disease
In the male	—	Breast enlargement (atrophy of testicles and loss of libido via gonadotrophin suppression and androgen lack)
		(Hazards of oestrogen treatment are discussed in Chapter 13)

Puberty is initiated by a reduction in this sensitivity and the consequent release of gonadotrophin releasing hormone. This causes the secretion of gonadotrophins causing stimulation of the ovaries. The earliest signs of puberty are the appearance of breast 'buds' and traces of pubic hair. The stages and timing of puberty including the establishment of menstruation (menarche) have been defined by Tanner (see further reading) and are shown in Fig. 12.2. The changes in the nipples are distinct. In stages 2 and 3 they enlarge and become pigmented. In stage 4 they form a dome-shaped projection above the breast but in stage 5, when the breast is fully mature, the areolae recede and become level with the surrounding skin and only the papillae remain projecting.

AGEING—THE MENOPAUSE

The function of the ovary begins to decline at about the age of 40 years and fertility diminishes from then onwards, although the menstrual cycle is maintained. The final failure of the ovaries happens relatively suddenly during one or two years in which the maturation of the follicles becomes infrequent and then ceases. The menses become less frequent or irregular and then stop but occasional ovulation may continue for a few months. A few years before the menopause oestrogen secretion from the ovaries begins to diminish and this decline continues afterwards until secretion virtually ceases. Thereafter oestrogen levels are maintained (in many women at substantial levels) by steroids de-

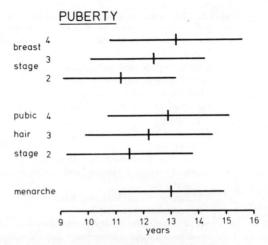

FIG. 12.2. The timing of female puberty. Each horizontal line includes 94% of all
normals, i.e. 3% are earlier and 3% are later. Vertical lines show the age at which
50% of normal girls have reached that stage of development.

rived from the adrenals. The cause of the ovarian failure is unknown
but it appears to be a primary process in the gonad. There is an
immediate response by the anterior pituitary so that the level of plasma
FSH rises to about ten times the premenopausal figure and the level of
plasma LH increases about two-fold.

Consequences of the menopause

Symptoms
The recent changes in social behaviour and relationships between the
sexes have been accompanied by greatly increased attention to the
menopause and its treatment. Many symptoms have been ascribed to
the menopause but some are much better defined than others.

'Hot flushes'
Over 90% of women get these at about the time the menses stop. The
flushes continue for two to three years, after which they become less
frequent and then cease. The typical 'hot flush' is heralded by an
unpleasant sensation followed by a feeling of warmth in the skin of the
face and upper chest. There is visible flushing and sweating which
persist for a few minutes. The 'flush' can come at any time and may
even wake the woman from sleep. Their frequency varies in individuals
from one to over twenty times a day and may become a serious embarrassment. The cause appears to be a vasomotor instability related to
the relatively abrupt fall in levels of oestrogens.

Mental symptoms

Although many symptoms such as tiredness, depression and irritability have been ascribed to the menopause they are not characteristic, affect a smaller proportion of women than 'hot flushes' and are less constantly related in time to the cessation of the menses. Nevertheless, many women pass through a time of several years in which they feel less well and during which the inevitable changes of age and home situations may be particularly hard to bear.

Vaginitis

One of the most troublesome objective results of the menopause is a reduction in cervical and vaginal secretions with atrophy of the vaginal mucosa. These changes cause dyspareunia and may predispose to vaginal infections.

In respect of *general health* the two most serious consequences of reduction in levels of oestrogens are deterioration in the arteries and skeleton. It seems that until the menopause oestrogens have a protective effect on the arterial intima and/or clotting systems so that the incidence of occlusive arterial disease, particularly in the heart, is much lower in middle-aged women than in men. After the menopause the incidence rises gradually until in later life it is approximately equal in the two sexes. Bone density is maintained in both sexes until middle life but thereafter gradually but continuously declines. This process is somewhat more rapid in women due presumably to their more abrupt loss of sex steroid secretion. A troublesome minor problem is slowly increasing hirsutes of the upper lip and face.

Sexual activity

After the menopause, sexual activity slowly declines, but its pattern and relation to levels of androgens and oestrogens have received less attention than this important topic warrants. It seems that libido and the capacity for orgasm are relatively well preserved, independent of oestrogen levels, particularly if the woman has had a satisfactory sex life before and is not subjected to major mental stress.

Management

The management of the menopause and concurrent symptoms, particularly with hormone replacement treatment ('HRT') has rightly received increasingly sympathetic attention in recent years. Many understandings both old and new about the menopause are under scrutiny but there is a lack of controlled data.

Oestrogens have a distinct action in reducing hot flushes but their effect on other menopausal symptoms is less certain and considerable placebo responses have been recorded. Vaginitis can be helped by local or systemic oestrogens. The value of long-term oestrogen treatment to prevent osteoporosis and improve general health not established and its safety is in some doubt. The following policy seems a reasonable compromise:

1. If hot flushes and general symptoms are not troublesome systemic oestrogens should be avoided. Vaginitis should be treated with local oestrogens.
2. If hot flushes are troublesome systemic oestrogens may be used.
3. If general symtoms predominate reassurance and sympathy are important; short courses of psychotropic drugs for depression may be indicated. If symptoms persist systemic oestrogens may be tried.
4. Systemic oestrogens are contra-indicated if the woman is over 60, has a history of ischaemic heart disease, venous or arterial thrombosis or malignant disease of the breast.
5. Systemic oestrogens should be given for a limited period of time only and three to five years is prudent. (Details of treatment schedules and precautions are given below.)

ASSESSMENT OF OVARIAN FUNCTION

Hormones

Measurements of plasma oestradiol and progesterone provide the best tests of ovarian hormone secretion. The results must be related to the stage of the menstrual cycle at which the specimen was taken (see Chapter 13). The ovarian response to gonadotrophin may be studied but these tests are not in routine use. The relationship between ovarian oestrogen production and pituitary LH secretion is less close than the comparable situation involving androgens, so that LH levels are a poor guide to ovarian function.

Follicles and corpus luteum

The simplest test for ovulation is the basal temperature chart (Fig. 12.3). The patient takes and charts her temperature every morning on waking throughout at least three menstrual cycles. One or two days after ovulation the temperature rises by about $0 \cdot 5°$ and persists at the higher level until the onset of menstruation. A well-defined rise in tem-

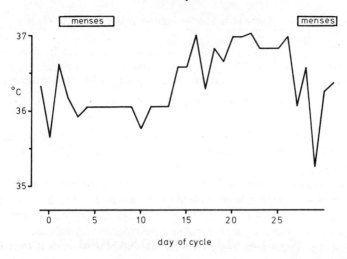

Fig. 12.3. A normal basal temperature chart showing an ovulatory rise on the 14th day.

perature is excellent evidence of ovulation, but an indefinite chart is not helpful because the rise may be absent in normal ovulatory cycles. The sequence of ovulation and corpus luteum formation may be demonstrated by changes in plasma oestradiol and progesterone. A full investigation is laborious and expensive but a single high value for progesterone three weeks after the end of menstruation indicates corpus luteum formation. An endometrial biopsy showing the secretory phase has the same significance. There are various radiological and ultrasonic techniques for demonstrating the size of the ovaries but laparoscopy is better; a ruptured follicle or corpus luteum may be demonstrated and a biopsy is taken. The management of specific clinical states is discussed below.

DISEASES OF THE OVARY

Tumours

Ovarian tumours are common but the large majority do not secrete hormones. Usually the functioning tumours are benign; the main types are in Table 12.2. The androgen secreting tumours cause virilisation. Those producing oestrogen or chorionic gonadotrophin present most commonly with partial precocious puberty.

TABLE 12.2. Functioning ovarian tumours

Hormone produced	Name of tumour	Comment
Oestrogen	Granulosa-theca cell	–
Androgen	Arrhenoblastoma	Commonest virilising adrenal tumour
	Gonadoblastoma	–
	Hilar cell	–
	Adrenal cell	From cell rests
Chorionic gonadotrophin	Teratoma	Malignant
Thyroxine	Teratoma	Benign

(Hormone secretion may be mixed; the principal one is shown)

FEMALE HYPOGONADISM

The classification of ovarian defects is incomplete and unsatisfactory. Also, the pathological and clinical groupings are often discordant.

Primary
The clinical features are related to the age at which the defect occurs.

Early (i.e. pre-pubertal)
Normal pre-pubertal ovaries are virtually never damaged by disease and defects are due to a failure of development leading to a 'streak' ovary or a hypoplastic one. This is called '*gonadal dysgenesis*'. The name 'Turner's syndrome' may be used also but the exact terminology is debatable.

Clinical
The condition is characterised by slow growth, a failure of puberty and the presence of other congenital anomalies. Occasionally the diagnosis

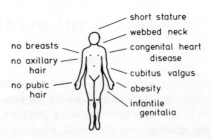

FIG. 12.4. Delayed puberty and associated anomalies in ovarian dysgenesis.

is suspected at birth because of some congenital anomaly or lymph-oedema of the extremities. Many different abnormalities have been recorded with ovarian dysgenesis but probably the commonest are a short neck with 'webbing', shield chest, cubitus valgus (increased 'carrying angle') and congenital heart disease, including coarctation of the aorta (Fig. 12.4). At puberty most patients are of short stature, somewhat overweight, with normal mentality but no secondary sexual characteristics. The uterus is small and the external genitalia infantile.

Aetiology
Rarely, no cause for the ovarian hypoplasia can be found but nearly all the patients have abnormalities of the sex chromosomes. About three-quarters of the patients are chromatin negative with a 45X karyotype. The remainder have various types of mosaicism (see Chapter 11) and consequently are chromatin positive to varying degrees.

Diagnosis
The demonstration of the abnormal karyotype is the most important single test. If the girl has passed the age of normal puberty, serum gonadotrophins, particularly FSH, are elevated but all other endocrine function is normal, including growth hormone secretion. In the younger child there is no hormonal abnormality at all—ovarian stimulation tests might be abnormal but are probably not justified. In the rare patient with apparently normal chromosomes a laparotomy or laparoscopy may be necessary to examine and biopsy the ovaries.

Treatment
The patient and her relatives may need considerable sympathy and support at first but usually the situation is soon accepted. It must be made clear that fertility is impossible. Replacement treatment with cyclical oestrogen and progestogen is indicated to produce an apparently normal puberty (see below for dosage). There is some uncertainty as to the age at which treatment should be started. If too early, there is at least a theoretical risk of reducing eventual adult height by epiphyseal fusion. If too late, psychological problems may be induced by delay in puberty. Somewhere between 14 and 16 years is reasonable, depending on the wishes of the patient and parents. Long-term treatment until the age of the natural menopause is indicated probably to protect against premature osteoporosis, but some patients get bored and discontinue treatment. This is followed by only slow regression of breasts and pubic hair.

Late-onset

The normal menopause of course comes into this category. Sometimes there is, for no apparent reason, even as early as the twenties, a *premature menopause*. The diagnosis is suggested by a high level of plasma FSH and confirmed, if necessary, by ovarian biopsy. The ovaries may be destroyed by surgery or radiation and, very rarely, infection or neoplasia. It seems that the equivalent of virus orchitis does not occur in the ovaries.

Primary ovarian dysfunction

There are many patients in whom it appears that there is a primary dysfunction of the ovaries, although it is suspected that faults in gonadotrophin secretion may be responsible. The defect falls short of ovarian failure and, although oestrogen production is maintained, the cyclical maturation of follicles is disturbed leading to irregular and/or anovulatory cycles. It is likely that there are a number of such conditions but they are poorly classified and the ovarian histology is variable. The best documented variety of ovarian dysfunction is the 'polycystic ovary' or 'Stein–Leventhal' syndrome, but even this is disputed. The syndrome is characterised by oligomenorrhoea or amenorrhoea, infertility, hirsutism (see Chapter 9) and iliac fossa pain. Obesity and virilisation may occur also but the clinical features are variable. The ovaries are enlarged with a smooth grey-white surface. Histologically, there is a thickened tunica albuginea, subcapsular fibrosis and multiple follicular cysts, some of which may be large. There are numerous atretic follicles and the theca interna is hyperplastic. The cyst fluid contains abnormal steroids. The biochemical changes are disputed but plasma androgens are slightly elevated and plasma LH is high also. The LH response to releasing hormone is high as in the normal luteal phase. It seems prudent to base the diagnosis on ovarian histology. In a considerable proportion of patients pregnancy has followed treatment with clomiphene but there is no long-term relief of the other features of the syndrome. Surgical wedge resection of the ovaries is going out of fashion. Treatment with suppressing doses of corticosteroids and/or cyclical oestrogen and progestogen has been recommended by some.

Secondary ovarian dysfunction

This term implies ovarian disorder due to defects in gonadotrophin secretion. The conditions present as a failure of puberty or a fault in later life with secondary oligomenorrhoea or amenorrhoea and/or infertility. Sometimes there is an associated general pituitary defect or virilisation.

Pituitary suppression
Causes are:

Androgen secreting tumour of ovary or adrenal. This produces clinical features of virilisation with clitoral hypertrophy, hirsutism and atrophy of breasts and uterus, as well as amenorrhoea.

Administration of androgens or anabolic steroids.

Adrenogenital syndrome (see Chapter 9). Usually this is apparent at birth but in a few patients there is a partial defect which is not apparent in infancy and may possibly be acquired rather than congenital. The presentation is with primary amenorrhoea and some degree of virilisation.

With endocrinopathies. Secondary amenorrhoea is common in Cushing's disease, due perhaps to suppression of gonadotrophin by adrenal androgens. Abnormal levels of thyroid function affect the ovaries. Infertility is usual in hyperthyroidism and menorrhagia may be a prominent feature in hypothyroidism.

Failure of gonadotrophin secretion panhypopituitarism
(See Chapter 8.) Any of the many disorders of the pituitary and hypothalamus which produce a general failure of the secretion of anterior pituitary hormones will cause ovarian failure. The clinical features are dominated by the other hormone deficiencies, particularly GH in children causing short stature, and TSH in adults causing secondary hypothyroidism.

Pituitary dysfunction
There are many circumstances in which the release of gonadotrophins is impaired, presumably in most instances due to defects in hypothalamic functions.
Causes include:

Psychogenic: depression, emotional stress, anorexia nervosa
Obesity
Major physical disease
Post-oral contraceptives
Cerebral tumours.

(For further discussion see Chapter 13).

DELAYED PUBERTY

This condition means a failure of development of the secondary sexual characteristics as well as a failure of menarche (the onset of menstruation). Primary amenorrhoea as a clinical problem is discussed in Chapter 13. Causes of delayed puberty include:

'Constitutional': may be familial and may be associated with less than average height; eventual sexual development normal

Low body weight

General Chronic Disease—e.g. asthma and coeliac disease

Ovarian dysgenesis

Pituitary insufficiency, including panhypopituitarism and isolated gonadotrophin deficiency

Rare syndromes, including the adrenogenital syndrome.

Management

The first step is to compare the girl's age and stage of sexual development with normal data (see further reading and Fig. 12.2) and also the height with charts of normal growth (Chapter 8). A pelvic examination may confirm the presence of a uterus.

No test can predict the onset of puberty so a flexible approach is necessary. A possible plan of action is as follows.

1. If puberty is in fact not retarded beyond the 3rd percentile in a girl of normal height without physical abnormality, reassurance and continued observation are correct.

2. If puberty is delayed, investigations are indicated even in the absence of physical abnormality; accompanying short stature is particularly significant and suggests ovarian dysgenesis or pituitary fault. Essential investigations are chromosome analysis and skull x-ray with plasma gonadotrophin, corticosteroid and thyroxine assays. Laparoscopy may be indicated.

3. If there is no evidence of a primary ovarian defect and gonadotrophins are low, a LHRH test may show a pituitary response, in which case the delayed puberty is probably constitutional.

4. If all investigations are negative, there is uncertainty as to when puberty should be induced with cyclical oestrogens/progestogens. If the girl is short there is a theoretical risk that early treatment may limit adult height by causing epiphyseal fusion. It is not known whether early treatment will interfere with a normal later puberty delayed for constitutional reasons. However, postponing treatment may cause

psychological problems for the girl and anxiety for the parents, so that precise rules cannot be made and each patient needs separate consideration. In constitutional delay, treatment will probably have to be given between 15 and 16 years, but if a permanent defect is found, puberty may be induced earlier, particularly if height is normal.

PRECOCIOUS PUBERTY

There are two forms, *complete* and *partial*.

Complete
This implies a full normal puberty with growth spurt, advanced bone age and the establishment of the menses. It can be produced only via a normally cyclical hypothalamic-pituitary axis.
Causes are:

'Idiopathic': much the commonest, and a relatively common occurrence in girls
Hypothalamic hamartomas
Hydrocephalus and other cerebral disorders
Weil-Albright syndrome: associated polyostotic fibrous dysplasia of bone and patchy skin pigmentation
Hypothyroidism.

Partial
This implies the development of secondary sexual characteristics, accelerated skeletal development and perhaps irregular uterine bleeding, but not cyclical menses.
Causes are:

Exogenous oestrogens (in error)
Oestrogen secreting tumour of ovary or adrenal (rare)
Gonadotrophin secreting tumour (rare).

Management
Comparison with normal ranges (Fig. 12.2) will show whether puberty is premature or not. If premature, investigation is necessary. A family history may be important, and physical examination should seek evidence of virilisation and an ovarian or adrenal tumour. X-ray of the skull is important. If an underlying cause is found, treatment is related to that. 'Constitutional' precocious puberty should be treated to con-

trol the obvious psychological problems and to increase eventual height by retarding epiphyseal fusion. Drugs to suppress gonadotrophin secretion are given. Medroxyprogesterone acetate has been most widely employed but danazol may be better.

OESTROGEN THERAPY

This may be used in three ways:

1. For replacement in ovarian failure; congenital, inflicted or normal menopausal.
2. For contraception or menstrual regulation.
3. Pharmacologically (i.e. in larger doses).

The hazards of the use of oestrogens as contraceptives have been well explored (see Chapter 13) but whether the same dangers exist when oestrogens are given in replacement doses is uncertain. Large doses of oestrogens carry an increased risk of pulmonary embolism.

Which oestrogen?

It has been claimed that 'natural' oestrogens (e.g. conjugated equine oestrogen) are safer than others but this is not proved and the preparations are expensive.

Stilboestrol is not recommended, mainly because it causes pigmentation of the nipples. The best preparation is ethinyl oestradiol in an oral dose of 10–30 mg a day, increased for some patients to 50 mg a day.

Schedules and precautions

For the premenopausal patient it is best to give cyclical treatment with an oestrogen/progestogen mixture and the oral contraceptive preparations are convenient for this (Chapter 13). The blood pressure should be checked twice a year but it is not known whether other routine examinations such as endometrial biopsy are necessary—such tests are not current practice.

For the post-menopausal patient cyclical combined oestrogen/progestogen is recommended with the progestogen included during days 7–13 of the cycle. There are commercial preparations in convenient packs which meet this requirement. The British Gynaecological Cancer Group (see further reading) consider that post-menopausal oestrogen therapy does carry some increased risk of endometrial cancer and recommend an endometrial biopsy every two years and immediate curettage if irregular bleeding should occur.

If the patient has no uterus then continuous oestrogen therapy may be given. In all patients regular blood pressure and breast examination are desirable.

It is sometimes claimed that androgens in small doses are helpful also in menopausal therapy but this is debatable.

Implants of the various hormones can be used but are not generally recommended. Local application of oestrogen containing creams (e.g. Dienoestrol $0 \cdot 01\%$) is valuable treatment for oestrogen-deficiency vaginitis but should not be applied elsewhere and is certainly not effective as a breast developer.

FURTHER READING

BEARD R.J. (Ed) (1976). *The Menopause*. MTP Press Ltd., Lancaster.

BRITISH GYNAECOLOGICAL CANCER GROUP (1981) Oestrogen replacement and endometrial cancer. *Lancet, i,* 1359.

JAMES V.H.T. *et al* (Eds) (1976). *The Endocrine Function of the Human Ovary*. Academic Press, London.

LEADER (1980) Fatness, puberty and ovulation. *New England Journal of Medicine,* **303,** 42.

PORTER R. & WHELAN J. (1979). *Sex, Hormones and Behaviour*. Excerpta Medica, Amsterdam.

STYNE D.M. & KAPLAN S.L. (1979). Normal and abnormal puberty in the female. *Pediatric Clinics of North America,* **26,** 123.

WATTEVILLE de H. (Ed) (1975). *Diagnosis and Treatment of Ovarian Neoplastic Alterations*. Excerpta Medica, Amsterdam.

YEN S.C.C (1980). The polycystic ovary syndrome. *Clinical Endocrinology,* **12,** 177.

Chapter 13
Gynaecological Endocrinology

The endocrine aspects of gynaecology and obstetrics are already important and likely to become more so. This text cannot deal with general gynaecological and obstetric theory and management but presents an outline of the hormonal physiology and the more important practical endocrine considerations.

NORMAL MENSTRUAL CYCLE

Many of the hormonal and histological changes of the cycle have now been defined and their relationships can be appreciated. The control of the cycle depends on a complex pattern of negative and positive feedback responses and it seems that follicle maturation is of prime importance. It is conventional to time the cycle from the onset of the menstrual flow.

A simplified and idealised display of the main events are shown in Fig. 13.1.

There are four phases:

Menstrual phase. During menstruation a number of ovarian follicles begin to mature through a complex series of histological changes.

194

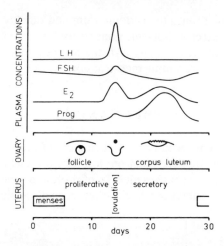

FIG. 13.1. The timing of the main events during the menstrual cycle. For clarity
the graphs of the plasma concentrations of the hormones have been separated
and only proportional changes are shown. LH = luteinising hormone, FSH
= follicle stimulating hormone, E_2 = oestradiol and Prog = progesterone.

Follicular phase. Further evolution of the follicles leads to the formation of several Graafian follicles but most of these then regress (atresia)
leaving (usually) a solitary follicle ready for ovulation. During the
maturation of the follicles, oestrogen production rises and also the
plasma level. The endometrium proliferates and the cervical mucus
increases in amount and viscosity. The rising oestrogen tends to
supress FSH release but with the final increase in size of the surviving
Graafian follicle there is a further increase in oestrogen production.
There seems to be a critical level at which oestrogens increase the
sensitivity of the gonadotrophs of the anterior pituitary to LHRH and
there is a sudden surge of LH release accompanied by a smaller rise in
FSH.

Ovulation phase. The LH surge causes rupture of the Graafian follicle
and ovulation.

Luteal phase. As the corpus luteum develops progesterone levels rise
and the endometrium becomes secretory in type. Towards the end of
the luteal phase the corpus luteum starts to regress, and it is presumably the consequent fall in progesterone which causes necrosis of the
endometrium and the onset of menstruation.

Implantation. If fertilisation of the ovum takes place the developing oocyte may implant into the endometrium and quickly forms the tro-phoblast. This secretes chorionic gonadotrophin which has properties similar to LH and therefore supports the corpus luteum and progester-one secretion, thus preventing menstruation.

PREGNANCY

Some of the more marked hormonal changes of pregnancy are shown in Fig. 13.2; they are dependent on hormone production by the 'feto-placental unit'. These changes must be of profound general importance during pregnancy but six practical aspects need discussion.

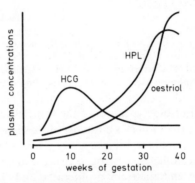

Fig. 13.2. Plasma hormone concentrations during pregnancy. The curves show the timing and proportional changes for each hormone but there are large indi-vidual variations. The scales are arbitrary. HPL = human placental lactogen and HCG = human chorionic gonadotrophin.

Pregnancy diagnosis. All the tests in general use depend on the de-tection of chorionic gonadotrophin in the urine. The tests become positive about six weeks after the beginning of the last menstrual period.

As early morning urine is more concentrated it is preferred as giving a more reliable result but this is not essential. The chorionic gonadotro-phin is detected by a simple slide or tube test utilising the agglutination of inert particles (e.g. latex) in connection with an antigen/antibody reaction.

Endocrine disease in pregnancy. This is dealt with in the appropriate chapters. The general point is that the high oestrogen level of preg-nancy increases the synthesis of hormone carrying globulins by the liver and therefore the levels of circulating hormones. This must be allowed for in the interpretation of endocrine tests during pregnancy.

Feto-placental nutrition. Measurement of plasma levels of oestriol during pregnancy is used to monitor the well-being of the fetus and thus to aid obstetric decisions. In general, low levels or a sudden fall are danger signals.

Management of pathological pregnancy. Sensitive methods for measuring chorionic gonadotrophin are valuable in determining whether a hydatidiform mole has been completely evacuated and also in early detection of choriocarcinoma. Further developments in the assays may permit other conclusions regarding the presence of early conception and early threatened abortion.

Habitual abortion. Attempts have been made to treat this condition with sex hormones to support the pregnancy during a supposed hormonal deficiency. Treatment during the first half of pregnancy may be hazardous to female fetuses. Particular associations are oestrogens with later genital adenocarcinoma in the child, and progestogen or androgen with variable masculinisation of the fetal external genitalia. These hazards and the lack of convincing evidence of benefit from the treatment has led to oestrogen therapy being abandoned for this purpose and progestogens being used only rarely.

Parturition. The hormonal events which may control the onset and course of labour are poorly understood but oxytocin does not seem to be essential. Discussion of the indications for the induction of labour is beyond the present text but in addition to surgical procedures use may be made of intravenous infusions of oxytocin. Prostaglandins by various routes are being used also but side-effects may be troublesome.

THE BREAST AND LACTATION

Development. During fetal life the primordial breast tissue is subjected to a different hormonal environment in the two sexes which may to some extent determine later development. Before puberty the nipples and potential breast tissue appear similar in both sexes. During puberty in the male there is usually no change but some enlargement of the nipples and/or breast tissue is common (Chapter 10); this regresses after a few years. Later enlargement can occur from the action of oestrogen. In the female it takes one to three years for the breasts to assume the fully adult form. Presumably oestrogens are important, acting with a suitable combination of several hormones.

Adult life. The breasts increase in volume during the menstrual cycle with a reduction after menstruation. A similar smaller change occurs in women taking oral contraceptives and an exaggerated response with discomfort (mastalgia or mastodynia) occurs in the pre-menstrual syndrome.

Size. Adult human female breasts vary widely in size and often are somewhat asymmetrical. In recent decades there has been a distinct increase in the average size of breasts related perhaps to greater height and earlier menarche. Marked deviations from the average in both directions are unfashionable leading to emotional distress and requests for medical aid. There is no reliable hormonal means of reducing breast size but if there is extreme enlargement, plastic surgery may be indicated. The medical treatment of small breasts is unsatisfactory also. Systemic oestrogens may produce slight increase but the results are hardly good enough to justify the risk. Local oestrogen creams are useless. Some enlargement may occur as a consequence of taking oral contraceptives. Plastic surgery may be indicated.

Pregnancy. During pregnancy the breasts enlarge under the combined influence of placental lactogen, oestrogen and progesterone. At first there is a proliferation of duct tissue and later an increase in secretory activity.

Lactation. The hormonal events which induce lactation are complex but pituitary prolactin is important. True milk production is established about two days after delivery. Continued lactation is dependent on suckling which initiates the milk ejection reflex, and maintains prolactin secretion. With continued suckling, lactation can go on for years, and during this time the raised prolactin levels to some extent depress ovulation and fertility.

Suppression of lactation. If there is no suckling, lactation fails after a few days but in the meantime distension of the breasts may cause discomfort. Treatment with analgesia may suffice. Oestrogens are contra-indicated because of the danger of thrombosis. Bromocriptine is safe and effective.

GALACTORRHOEA

The secretion of milk from non-puerperal female breasts is not uncommon but often the secretion is slight and easily overlooked. A large number of causes have been recorded but only the five commoner types will be discussed here. Prolactin assays provide the opportunity to determine some of the hormonal mediation of the various types. It is evident that high levels of prolactin do not always cause galactorrhoea and that galactorrhoea can occur in the presence of normal levels of prolactin.

Pituitary tumours. Many kinds have been implicated but the most important is the *prolactinoma* (prolactin secreting adenoma, usually chromophobe). A number of previously termed 'non-secreting' adenomas are of this type. The plasma prolactin is raised and the treatment is that of the tumour although bromocriptine (see below) may be used.

Hypothalamic. The aetiology is presumed to involve the hypothalamus but some of the patients have microadenomas of the anterior pituitary which become manifest years later. Usually, the clinical features include secondary amenorrhoea or infertility. Levels of plasma prolactin are raised but can be suppressed by bromocriptine, often with restoration of fertility.

In association with endocrine disease. Many associations have been reported including various organic brain lesions, ectopic hormone secretion and adrenal disease. The best known association is with hyper- and hypo-thyroidism.

Neurogenic. This type may be induced by many conditions of the chest wall including thoracotomy, mastectomy, trauma, stimulation of the breast and herpes zoster.

Drug induced. As well as in association with the administration of sex hormones, galactorrhoea may occur with the use of many psychotrophic drugs. The phenothiazines, tricyclic antidepressants, haloperidol and anxiolytics have all been implicated. Reserpine and methyl dopa may cause it also. Most of these drugs stimulate prolactin secretion, some by acting as dopamine antagonists.

Management

The discovery of a cause among those above may indicate appropriate treatment. It is particularly important to seek a pituitary tumour. In the 'hypothalamic' form various hormone treatments have been tried with partial success. Pregnancy following clomiphene has resulted in remission. For patients with raised plasma prolaction, bromocriptine in an oral dose of 2·5 mg one to three times a day is likely to be satisfactory—the patient must be warned that the treatment may restore fertility.

DYSMENORRHOEA

Pain in the lower abdomen or nearby, just before the onset or during the first one or two days of menstruation, is a common complaint in young women. It may be accompanied by heavy blood loss and irregular menses. Very occasionally, organic pelvic disease may be present but there is no recognised hormonal abnormality. Most patients control the symptoms with analgesics but occasionally the condition is disabling. Ovulation seems to be a prerequisite and its suppression with oral contraceptives will give relief in most patients as well as regulating the menses and reducing blood loss. The hazards of this treatment are discussed below.

PREMENSTRUAL SYNDROME (CYCLICAL OEDEMA)

A large proportion of women notice physical or mental changes during the cycle, particularly in the week or so before the menses. Usually the symptoms are trivial but sometimes they are more severe and lead to a request for treatment. Rarely, the condition is disabling. The commonest features are weight gain due to water retention with swelling of fingers, feet and abdomen, breast engorgement and discomfort, migraine and changes in mood with nervous tension or depression. The symptoms are relieved with the onset of menstruation.

There is no known hormonal basis for the syndrome. Supression of ovulation, and therefore of luteal secretion of progesterone does not help. No hormonal manipulation has been generally successful but progestogens may help. Diuretics are useful to control the oedema. Sometimes mastalgia is the presenting symptom and of considerable severity. If examination shows no evidence of localised breast disease, bromocriptine or danazol may be given with benefit to some patients.

DYSFUNCTIONAL UTERINE BLEEDING

Changes in the pattern of the menstrual cycle with heavy menstrual loss (menorrhagia), intermittent bleeding (metrorrhagia), frequent bleeding (polymenorrhoea) or infrequent bleeding (oligomenorrhoea) are common symptoms throughout reproductive life, but particularly at puberty and towards the menopause. The causes are numerous but it is helpful to distinguish the so-called 'organic' from the 'dysfunctional'. The former are those in which there is local disease of the pelvic organs or a generalised physical disease, while the latter implies a hormonal abnormality, usually with ovulation. The first and essential step is to exclude 'organic' causes of which the major types are:

Benign and malignant pelvic tumours
Pelvic sepsis
Complications of pregnancy
Systemic disease such as blood dyscrasias.

Uterine curettage may be indicated, particularly in the perimenopausal patient. If 'organic' causes have been excluded, 'dysfunctional' bleeding is diagnosed by exclusion. The main causes are:

1. Hypothalamic/pituitary: Puberty
                           Obesity and malnutrition
                           Psychogenic
                           Tumours, etc.
2. Ovarian: Menopause
            Polycystic disease
            Tumours
3. Drugs: Steroids
          Psychotropic
4. Thyroid and adrenal dysfunction

In most instances, history and physical examination will suffice to reach a working diagnosis but sometimes investigation will be necessary. A basal temperature chart may help to detect ovulation—a suitably timed measurement of plasma progesterone may detect a corpus luteum.

Chapter 13

Treatment
If fertility is not desired and the patient is pubertal or peri-menopausal, reassurance and delay is usually appropriate. If the cycle is anovulatory, heavy loss may be terminated by giving a progestogen such as norethisterone. Sometimes, oestrogen is effective. Later, the timing and magnitude of menstruation can be controlled by cyclical administration of an oestrogen/progestogen preparation. If fertility is desired, the induction of ovulation with antioestrogen may be appropriate.
N.B. It is most important not to use hormonal treatment thoughtlessly and overlook a correctable or dangerous primary cause of irregular bleeding.

PRIMARY AMENORRHOEA

This term indicates the failure of the onset of menstruation. All but 3% of normal girls should have begun to menstruate by the age of 15 years so that delay beyond this age merits investigation. Some of the causes have been discussed in other chapters but the following classification is helpful.

With normal secondary sexual characteristics. This situation implies normal oestrogen production and probably normal total gonadotrophin secretion. Many of the patients will have no detectable abnormality and will develop normal menses later. In a few patients gynaecological examination will show an anatomical fault such as an imperforate hymen, vaginal agenesis and/or uterine agenesis.

With normal breast development but no pubic or axillary hair. This rare combination is likely to be due to the bizarre condition called the testicular feminisation syndrome. These patients have normal male sex chromosomes (or rarely mosaics) with testes and normal male levels of testosterone. The condition is inherited and half the XY individuals in a family are likely to be affected. All the tissues are insensitive to androgens probably because of absent or defective receptor sites for androgen in the cytosol so that androgen is not transported to the nucleus. Female external genitalia are formed in the fetus and at birth the condition is unsuspected. At puberty, breast development occurs and female contours formed but body hair is scanty or absent. Otherwise, the patients appear to be entirely normal phenotypic females until examination reveals an incomplete vagina with absent uterus. The testes may be palpable in the groins. As the patient will have been reared as a girl, the testes should be removed (in addition they are liable to malignancy) and oestrogen treatment given to complete sexual development.

With no secondary sexual characteristics. About half these patients will have a primary gonadal fault and the others will have secondary hypogonadism due to a failure of gonadotrophin secretion (Chapter 8).

With ambiguous external genitalia. This rare situation is likely to be due to an adrenogenital syndrome, virilising tumour or true hermaphroditism.

SECONDARY AMENORRHOEA

This implies the partial (oligomenorrhoea) or complete failure of menstruation which had previously been established. Some of the causes have been discussed in Chapter 12. The following classification will help in management.

Pregnancy
This seemingly obvious condition is overlooked regularly, particularly in the young girl or older women, especially if the patient is obese.

Menopause
This is not likely to lead to difficulties in diagnosis particularly if menopausal symptoms are present. A spontaneous premature menopause, even as early as the twenties, is not rare. A high level of plasma FSH is confirmatory.

'Functional' defect of hypothalamus/pituitary
This is a common disorder with many causes.

Physiological. A transient defect of this kind should be regarded as normal during puberty and before the menopause.

Psychogenic. Any emotional stress such as school examinations, change of job or personal problems commonly leads to transient amenorrhoea.

Changes in body weight. A rapid rise or fall in body weight can suppress menstruation. With time the menses are likely to return, particularly if normal body weight is restored. The most striking example of this situation is anorexia nervosa where amenorrhoea is a cardinal feature. Prolonged physical exertion is relevant also.

Intercurrent disease. Any major physical disease may be complicated by amenorrhoea.

Endocrinopathies. Most endocrine disease can cause secondary amenorrhoea but it is particularly common in hyperthyroidism, severe diabetes and Cushing's syndrome.

Post oral contraceptive (see below).

'Organic' brain and pituitary disease
This includes various tumours, infections, infarctions and granulomas of the brain, para-pituitary and pituitary areas.

Pelvic disease. Of course surgical removal of the uterus and ovaries may be relevant but in addition inflammatory disease of the pelvic organs and endometrial adhesions may prevent menstruation.

With galactorrhoea
This may occur spontaneously, with a prolactin secreting pituitary tumour or after pregnancy.

INFERTILITY

At least 10% of marriages are infertile and this is a frequent cause of medical consultation. It is essential that both partners are examined before elaborate investigations are undertaken in either. A history should be taken to enquire about the menses and whether there has been any previous illness or treatment in either partner which might have damaged the gonads or pelvic organs. Discreet enquiries are made to confirm as far as possible that intercourse is normal and not unduly infrequent or inappropriately timed. If all seems well it is conventional to require twelve months of failure to conceive before investigations are indicated. The following sequence may then be followed:

1. Physical examination of both partners including search for general disease such as thyroid dysfunction or genital tract abnormalities. If negative, a basal temperature chart (Chapter 12) for at least three cycles and a sperm count should be obtained.

2. If the sperm count is confirmed to be low, investigations should be carried out on the male (Chapter 10).
3. If the sperm count is normal investigations should be carried out on the female.

Investigation

If there is evidence of ovulation, the next step is establishing the patency of the Fallopian tubes. If they are normal, there is little which can be achieved by further investigation and it is best to advise further attempts at conception with intercourse concentrated at the time of ovulation. Many women in these circumstances will conceive eventually.

If there is doubt about ovulation, or if there is oligomenorrhoea/amenorrhoea, endocrinological investigation is indicated. The presence of ovulation can be established by observing a single estimation of plasma progesterone above 16 nmol/l between the 18th and 26th day of the cycle.

Subsequent investigations can be of high complexity but it is desirable to seek:

An enlarged sella turcica
Hyperprolactinaemia
Changes in gonadotrophins, and,
Failure of LHRH response.

Treatment

There may be benefit from advice concerning incompetent intercourse, the treatment of general disease or the relief of tubal occlusion. Hormonal treatment may be of four kinds.

Cyclical oestrogen/progestogen. If there is oligomenorrhoea or amenorrhoea this treatment may be given for a few cycles to induce menstruation. After stopping the treatment it is hoped that the next cycle will be ovulatory and that the endometrium will be ready for implantation.

Clomiphene (and Tomoxifen). These substances are anti-oestrogens and cause the release of gonadotrophin presumably by increasing the sensitivity of the gonadotrophs in the anterior pituitary to endogenous LHRH. Clomiphene is preferred, and may be given in a dose of 50 mg per day by mouth for 5 days beginning on the 5th day of the cycle.

Intercourse must be concentrated about the 15th day. If conception does not occur repeat courses at progressively higher doses e.g. 100, 150, or 200 mg per day are given. If there are no natural menses, clomiphene may be started 5 days after the onset of bleeding induced by progestogen withdrawal (e.g. norethisterone 10 mg per day for 5 days). The conception rate after clomiphene is high. The spontaneous abortion rate is substantial but multiple pregnancies are uncommon and no serious adverse effects have been observed.

Gonadotrophin. If pituitary response is defective, ovulation can be induced sometimes by a combination of chorionic gonadotrophin (from human pregnancy urine) and pituitary FSH. Such treatment may result in spectacular multiple pregnancies and is expensive. Its use should be confined to special centres.

Bromocriptine. In patients with hyperprolactinaemia and the galactorrhoea/amenorrhoea syndrome, bromocriptine in a dose of 2.5 mg 1–3 times per day by mouth promptly suppresses the levels of prolactin to normal and permits normal ovulation.

HORMONAL CONTRACEPTIVES

Many methods of fertility control are available and to find the most appropriate method in various circumstances may need careful consideration. The present discussion is limited to hormonal contraceptives but it must not be assumed that they are always appropriate.

Combined oral contraceptives

These are now used by a substantial proportion of all fertile women so doctors in many different kinds of practice need to be aware of the actions and hazards of these preparations.

Chemistry and formulation
Combined oral contraceptives contain an oestrogen and a progestogen. The oestrogen is either:

Ethinyl oestradiol—20 to 50 mg per day
or
Mestranol   —   50 mg per day.

The progestogen is usually a 19–nortestosterone derivative, e.g.

Norethisterone	0.5 to 1.0	mg per day
Norethisterone acetate	1.0 to 4.0	mg per day
Ethynodiol diacetate	0.5 to 2.0	mg per day
1-Norgestrel	0.05 to 0.25	mg per day
Lynoestrenol	2.5	mg per day

There are many oral contraceptive pills available with various combinations and quantities of the hormones above. Most of the preparations contain the same dose in all the tablets but a few (called 'triphasic') have three different formulations which are taken in turn so that towards the end of the cycle the dose of oestrogen is lower while that of progestogen is higher, to mimic the normal sequence.

Efficacy and mode of action
With the possible exception of the lowest dose pills, all the available oral contraceptives are virtually 100% effective if taken regularly and even an occasional missed single dose does not matter; nearly all failures are due to non-compliance. The mode of action is still not wholly understood and it is not clear why an oestrogen/progestogen mixture is effective while each on its own is less so. Probably the major action is to suppress the normal mid-cycle peak of LH secretion and the consequent ovulation. Gonadotrophin secretion generally is reduced. In addition, there are changes in the cervical mucus and endometrium which also help to prevent pregnancy.

Prescribing
It is generally advised that 'the pill' should be supplied only after a medical consultation involving a full physical examination and speculum examination (and cervical smear). It is debatable whether this is necessary in the case of young women and there is a danger that this ritual may inhibit some girls, particularly young ones, from seeking contraceptive advice when they most need it. Regular review is recommended also and this is probably more important, particularly in the older woman. Oral contraceptives in this country are available only under medical supervision.

Method of administration
Treatment with a combined oral contraceptive is started on the fifth day of a menstrual cycle, day one being the onset of menstruation. (Triphasic pills are started on day one). The pill is taken as a single dose at the same time each day but without any fixed relationship to

meals. It is usual to take a pill for 21 days and then none for 7 days during which menstruation occurs. This is not essential (except for the triphasic pill) and it is possible to take 'the pill' continuously for long periods without additional ill effects, so far as is known. Manufacturers present 'the pill' in a variety of ingenious monthly packs to make it easier to remember to take it. Sometimes 7 days of inert tablets are included so that a pill is taken every day. Additional contraceptive precautions should be taken during the first two weeks of administration.

Age limits and duration of use
There is no lower age limit for the use of 'the pill'. It is not known whether prolonged use is specifically harmful or not; many women have now taken 'the pill' for ten years or more but obviously there must be doubt as to the safety of taking such a potent preparation over very long periods of time.

The small but significant mortality associated with taking oral contraceptives increases sharply after the age of 35 years so a change to an alternative method of contraception should be advised at that age.

Selection of patients
The 'pill' is very popular so that many clients select themselves. The prescribers role is to seek contra-indications by history and examination, and advise accordingly. A discussion of relative risks may be needed.

Absolute contra-indications. These are few and comprise present or past evidence of:

Liver disease—particularly jaundice or pruritus of pregnancy, recent
  infective hepatitis (6/12) and hereditary excretory defects
Carcinoma of the breast
Deep vein thrombosis with or without pulmonary embolus
Pulmonary hypertension
Vascular or neurological eye disease
Pituitary tumour
Pancreatitis
Homozygous sickle-cell disease

Relative contra-indications. Varicose veins
Fibroids
Hypertension
Hyperlipidaemia

Cigarette smoking—at all ages this increases the mortality associated with oral contraceptives by two to three fold. This effect is particularly important in women over 35.

(*N.B.* carcinoma of cervix or uterus is not a contra-indication.)

Selecting the appropriate 'pill'

It is best to be familiar with a small number of the many alternatives available. A suitable formulation to begin with for most young women is:

Ethinyl Oestradiol	30 mg
l-Norgestrel	150 mg

If the patient reacts unfavourably it may be necessary to change to another formulation and difficulties with bleeding are common but heavy bleeding, break-through bleeding and failure of withdrawal bleeding may all benefit from an increase in dose of progestogen; this may carry some penalty from an increased incidence of adverse reactions.

Drug interactions

Combined oral contraceptives may reduce the effectiveness of hypotensive drugs and coumarins. Concurrent administration of barbiturates, anticonvulsants, dichoralphenazone, phenylbutazone, rifampicin or ampicillin tends to reduce the effectiveness of oral contraceptives so that breakthrough bleeding and pregnancy may result.

Consequences

The more important consequences are considered under four headings, of quite different significance.

Side-effects. These are more or less unpleasant symptoms associated with taking the 'pill'—some may be placebo reactions.
   Headache
   Weight gain
   Bloating
   Mastalgia
   Acne
   Depression (?)
   Loss of libido
   Changes in bleeding
   Enlargement of fibroids.

Sometimes women will tolerate quite severe side-effects as the price of reliable contraception but sometimes the side-effects cause non-compliance and lead to unwanted pregnancy.

Often the side-effects can be eliminated or reduced by changing the formulation; a change to another method of contraception may be desirable but is not essential.

(*N.B.* Many women feel better when taking 'the pill' than when not— in particular headaches may be less and libido increased.)

Metabolic effects. Combined oral contraceptives produce many biochemical effects in addition to the hormonal alterations on which their effectiveness depends. Nearly all the changes are due to the oestrogen component. The changes are slight and do not cause any immediate or obvious illness (except as noted) but the direction of the changes are such as to suggest that they might damage health after many years. Hence the concern at the following:

  Deterioration in glucose tolerance
  Increase in plasma triglycerides (cholesterol?)
  Partial pyridoxine deficiency
  Partial folic acid deficiency (anaemia has been reported)
  Reduced prothrombin time
  Increased platelet aggregation
  (In addition, there is an increase in all the hormone binding proteins).

Adverse reactions. These are clinically evident failures of health which have been shown to have an increased incidence in 'pill' takers particularly after the age of 35. Usually, their occurrence means that combined oral contraceptives must be discontinued permanently.

  Vascular thrombosis, including deep vein thrombosis, pulmonary embolism, cerebral thrombosis and myocardial infarction.

  Jaundice
  Pancreatitis
  Hypertension
  Gallstones

It is important to place these adverse reactions in perspective. Thromboembolic disease occurs only once in about 1000 women years' of 'pill' taking. Overall, it has not been possible to show any increase of death rate in 'pill' takers. The occurrence of hypertension, which is not rare, is probably the main justification for follow-up examinations. There is no definite evidence of any increased risk of cancer.

Post oral contraceptive effects

Amenorrhoea after discontinuing 'the pill' is not uncommon but it is impossible to tell whether it would have occurred anyway. It is not certain whether fertility is slightly reduced or not; most women conceive readily when they wish to.

Other hormonal contraceptives

Progestogens may be used alone. There are several preparations with which an oral progestogen (e.g. norethisterone 350 mg per day) is taken continuously. Variable menstrual bleeding may be troublesome and the contraceptive action is slightly less than that of the combined preparations but the hazards are thought to be less.

A long-acting injectable progestogen can provide contraception for up to three months after a single dose; this preparation is not currently licensed for general use.

Benefits or oral contraceptives

Although many possible consequences of oral contraceptives have been outlined above, it is important to appreciate that serious side-effects are uncommon and the risk is, for example, much less than that of moderate cigarette smoking. The benefits from the reliability of oral contraceptives in terms of personal and social well-being out-weigh the hazards.

FURTHER READING

BAIRD D.T. (1979). Endocrinology of female infertility. *British Medical Bulletin*, **35**, 193.

BEARD R.J. (Ed) (1976). *The Menopause*. M.T.P. Press, Lancaster.

CROSIGNANI P.G. & MISHELL D.R. (Eds) (1977). *Ovulation in the Human*. Academic Press, London.

FRASER W.M. & BLACKARD W.G. (1975). Medical conditions that effect the breast and lactation. *Clinical Obstetrics and Gynecology*, **18** (2), 51.

GUILLEBAUD J. (1980). *The Pill*. O.U.P. Oxford.

HUTTON J.D. *et al*. (1979). Steroid endocrinology after the menopause; a review. *Journal of the Royal Society of Medicine*, **72**, 835.

PHILIPP E.E. & CARRUTHERS G.B. (1981). *Infertility*. Heinemann, London.

ROYAL COLLEGE OF GENERAL PRACTITIONERS (1981). Further analysis of mortality in oral contraceptive users. *Lancet, i*, 541.

SCOMMEGNA A. & DMOWSKI W.P. (1973). Dysfunctional uterine bleeding. *Clinical Obstetrics and Gynecology*, **16** (3) 221.

TIETZE C. & LEWIT S. (1979). Life risks associated with reversible methods of fertility regulation. *International Journal of Gynaecology & Obstetrics*, **16** (6), 456 (see rest of volume also).

Chapter 14
Miscellaneous Matters

CARCINOID SYNDROME

There is an uncommon group of tumours to which the term 'carcinoid' is applied. They arise from argentaffin cells and often contain silver staining granules. They may occur at any age but are commoner in older persons, equally in both sexes. The tumours have a malignant histological appearance but are slow growing. Most do not metastasise and are removed after chance discovery or local symptoms. When metastases do occur they grow slowly also but eventually are extensive and then general symptoms (the carcinoid syndrome) arise. They may occur anywhere in the gut and in the lung but 90% of carcinoid tumours are in the ileocaecal region (and rarely spread).

The symptoms and signs of the carcinoid syndrome may arise in several locations:

Vasomotor. The most characteristic feature is facial flushing. It may last for minutes or hours and be occasional or frequent. The flush may spread to the upper chest and elsewhere. There may be sweating, dizziness and hypotension.

Gut. Abdominal discomfort, sometimes with colic, nausea, vomiting and particularly diarrhoea, is common and may be recurrent or persistent.

Heart. In advanced cases there may be right heart endocardial fibrosis going on to pulmonary stenosis and right heart failure. Left-sided lesions are rare but have been recorded.

Chest. There may be intermittent changes in the depth and rate of respiration with episodes of acute bronchial asthma.

The biochemical basis of the generalised syndrome is that carcinoid tumours synthesise and secrete a variety of vasoreactive compounds. The pattern of synthesis depends to some extent on the location of the tumour and the cells from which it was derived, but particularly implicated are 5-hydroxytryptophan, 5-hydroxytryptamine, histamine and bradykinin. This suggests some similarity between carcinoid tumour and medullary carcinoma of the thyroid.

Diagnosis of the carcinoid syndrome rests on finding a high level of urinary 5-hydroxyindole acetic acid which is invariably present. Treatment is by removal of the tumour as far as possible but because of the nature of the condition radical cure is unlikely. Many drug treatments have been used with little success but α-adrenergic blocking drugs may usefully reduce the frequency of the flushing attacks.

MULTIPLE ENDOCRINE NEOPLASIA SYNDROMES

These conditions, also called the 'pluriglandular syndromes' are hereditary conditions transmitted as autosomal dominants in which an adenoma or adenomatosis occurs in two or more endocrine glands and in particular:

Pituitary adenoma—with or without hormone excess
Parathyroid adenoma
Insulinoma
Medullary carcinoma of thyroid
Phaeochromocytoma
Cushing's syndrome.

Many combinations have been reported. *Type I* comprises pituitary adenoma, islet cell tumour and hyperparathyroidism. *Type IIa* (or Sipple syndrome) comprises phaeochromocytoma, medullary carcinoma of thyroid and hyperparathyroidism. *Type IIb* or (or III) comprises phaeochromocytoma, medullary carcinoma of thyroid in combination with rare tumours. Many other associated tumours have been reported particularly in type I.

HORMONE SECRETING TUMOURS OF
NON-ENDOCRINE ORIGIN
(ECTOPIC HORMONE PRODUCTION)

Many neoplasms, particularly carcinomas, synthesise compounds which are inappropriate or unrelated to the tissue from which the tumour arose. This discussion is concerned mostly with such compounds, usually peptides, as are identical to hormones or so similar as to have the same biological actions. Sometimes, the amount of compound released is large and clinical features appear. It is unusual for a tumour to release more than one compound in quantity. This subject is of great theoretical interest and of increasing practical importance as more patients with the syndromes are identified, giving opportunities for treatment, even if only palliation, and the use of the hormones as tumour markers to guide management.

The clinical presentation may be dominated by other effects of the tumour. It is likely that many cases are not diagnosed because they occur in the terminal stages of malignant disease so that the true incidence is unknown. Sometimes the presentation is with the endocrine syndrome and there is the possibility of identifying a neoplasm at an early stage with consequent better prospect of cure. Some of the syndromes are identical with the usual endocrine disease but there are many exceptions and differences in detail as indicated below:

Inappropriate ADH secretion. The presentation is with changes in cerebral function due to water intoxication (Chapter 8). The clinical features are the same in those instances due to non-malignant cerebral or lung disease (in which case the ADH is coming presumably from the posterior pituitary) as in those where the ADH is being synthesised by a tumour.

Ectopic ACTH syndrome. This is due most commonly to an oat-celled carcinoma of the bronchus releasing large amounts of ACTH-like material accompanied usually by MSH. Although the levels of plasma 'ACTH' are high, indeed diagnostically higher than those in pituitary Cushing's disease, and the plasma cortisol is high also, the usual clinical features of Cushing's syndrome are lacking because the condition progresses too quickly for them to develop. Presentation is usually in a man with a rapid onset of oedema, pigmentation, weight loss, weakness and sometimes the symptoms of diabetes mellitus. Typically there is a hypokalaemic alkalosis. Adrenocortical enzyme inhibitors may be useful in treatment.

Hypoglycaemia. Symptomatic hypoglycaemia may be associated with carcinomas but is more commonly related to mesenchymal tumours, particularly large benign fibromas. The biochemical cause of the hypoglycaemia has not been proved. Glucose consumption by the tumour seems unlikely and it is probably that the tumours secrete compounds with insulin-like activity. If removal is impossible, streptozotocin which necroses β cells may be helpful.

Polycythaemia. This occurs as an increase in red cell mass without changes in other cells and without splenomegaly. The related malignant tumours are usually but not exclusively renal. Polycythaemia may occur also with benign renal tumours and hydronephrosis. It is likely that red cell production is increased because of the release of an erythropoietin—like material from the lesion.

Atypical carcinoid syndrome Non-carcinoid tumours may produce all the usual features of the carcinoid syndrome. The term 'atypical' refers to the tumours and perhaps some aspects of the biochemistry. Methyldopa may reduce some of the symptoms such as diarrhoea, but not the flushing.

Gynaecomastia and arthropathy Both these features, alone or together, are not uncommon in patients with carcinoma of the bronchus. There is doubt as to the hormones responsible but secretion of gonadotrophin and growth hormone from the tumours has been reported.

Hypercalcaemia. This is one of the commonest syndromes of metabolic derangement with malignant disease. In some patients bony metastases have led presumably to the release of calcium. The condition occurs also in the absence of apparent skeletal involvement and in these patients the biochemical mechanism is obscure. Attempts to find material like parathyroid hormone have been unsuccessful.

Miscellaneous. Other syndromes of ectopic hormone production have been found. Changes in thyroid function may occur in patients with trophoblastic tumours secreting gonadotrophin but clinical hyperthyroidism is not usually present and the involvement of TSH is uncertain. Long-standing hypophosphataemia and generalised bone disease has been noted with mesenchymal tumours and haemangiomas but the chemical mediator is unknown.

GASTROINTESTINAL HORMONES

Hormone secreting cells

The whole length of the GI tract from oesophagus to rectum contains a large number of hormone secreting cells and has been described as the largest endocrine gland. The cells are now often referred to as part of the APUD system, which is an acronym from the words Amine Precursor Uptake and Decarboxylation, describing two of their functions. The intestinal APUD cells lies in the mucosa. Microvilli project into the intestinal lumen from one end of the cells and there are secretory granules at the other. Presumably the cells respond to changes in the composition of the gut contents but there is response also to autonomic nervous stimuli in some instances. There is a specific type of cell producing each hormone and the types of cell have different distributions in the GI tract so that the hormones are produced at different levels but there is considerable overlap.

The hormones. These are polypeptides of about 20 to 40 amino acids in

TABLE 14.1. Some Gastro-intestinal Hormones

Hormone	Action	Location
Gastrin	Stimulates gastric acid secretion	Antrum, islets intestine
Cholecystokinin (CCK)	Stimulates gall bladder contraction and pancreatic enzyme secretion	Duodenum and jejunum
(All compounds in this group inhibit acidity and release insulin)		
Secretin	Stimulates pancreatic juice and bicarbonate secretion	Duodenum and jejunum
Glucagon	Releases insulin	Fundus, islets
Vasoactive intestinal peptide (VIP)	Relaxes smooth muscle; vasodilation and hypotension	?
Gastric inhibitory peptide (GIP)	Inhibits release of gastric acid	Intestine
Bombesin	Stimulates gastrin release	?
Pancreatic polypeptide (PP)	?	Pancreas
(Other probable GI hormones are motilin, neurotensin and somatostatin)		

length although some may be secreted as larger precursors and many fragments of the hormones retain some of the biological activity of the parent compounds. Many of the amino acid sequences are common to several hormones. Some of the best established hormones are listed in Table 14.1. Based on similarities of structure and function three main groups can be distinguished.

Physiology. Most of the actions of the GI hormones are on the gut and pancreas but their chemical relationship with the enkephalins and possible CNS effects are of particular interest.

Diseases. The best known conditions associated with excess of gut hormones are glucagonoma and gastrinoma, described elsewhere. VIP has been implicated in a syndrome of chronic diarrhoea and achlorhydria. The significance of GI hormones in general and gut disease remains to be determined.

HORMONAL TREATMENT OF CANCER

The treatment of cancer by drugs has been greatly extended in recent years and medical oncology has emerged as a clinical discipline. The relative values of radiotherapy, antimitotic drugs and hormonal manipulations are debatable—only some of the possible uses of the latter are listed here.

Leukaemias. Corticosteroids in large doses are included in most regimes of treatment, particularly if bleeding is troublesome.

Cerebral tumours. Corticosteroids may produce a short but useful remission of symptoms by reducing cerebral oedema.

Endometrial carcinoma. Surgery and radiotherapy are the major treatments but progestogens may retard the growth of the primary or secondary tumours.

Carcinoma of breast. About one third of breast cancers are hormone dependent to some extent but there is little consensus of opinion as to how this can be exploited. In the premenopausal woman, oophorectomy to reduce oestrogens is recommended. Sometimes adrenalectomy or hypophysectomy have led to remission of disseminated disease. After the menopause androgens, non-virilising androgens or anti-oestrogens are used widely. Although it seems paradoxical, oestrogen may be effective in older women.

Carcinoma of prostate. If there is extensive disease or obstruction oestrogens may help by causing some shrinkage of the tumour. Stilboestrol, 1 mg three times a day is a usual regime. Higher doses are not recommended because of the increased risk of thrombosis.

FURTHER READING

ALBERTS W.M. *et al*. (1980). Mixed multiple endocrine neoplasia syndromes. *Journal of the American Medical Association*, **244**, 1236.

BLOOM S.R. (1980). Gut and brain—endocrine connections. *Journal of the Royal College of Physicians*, **14**, 51.

BUCHANAN K.D. (Ed) (1979). Gastrointestinal hormones. *Clinics in Endocrinology and Metabolism*, **8** (2).

POGACH L.M. & VAITUKAITIS J.L. (1981). Ectopic production of pituitary hormones. In C. Beardwell & G.L. Robertson (Eds). The pituitary. *Clinical Endocrinology. Vol. I.* Butterworths, London.

Index